UNRAVELING > REWEAVING

Passing Through and Beyond Parkinson's

UNRAVELING > REWEAVING
Passing Through and Beyond Parkinson's

Claire Blatchford

Lorian Press LLC

Unraveling > Reweaving:
Passing Through and Beyond Parkinson's

CoverArt by Claire Blatchford
Book Design by Jeremy Berg

ISBN: 978-1-939790-49-1

Blatchford, Claire
Unraveling > Reweaving:
Passing Through and Beyond Parkinson's/Claire Blatchford

First Print Edition May 2021

Lorian Press LLC is a private, for profit business which publishes
works approved by the Lorian Association. Current titles can be
found at www.lorianpress.com.

The Lorian Association is a not-for-profit educational organization.
Its work is to help people bring the joy, healing, and blessing
of their personal spirituality into their everyday lives. This
spirituality unfolds out of their unique lives and relationships
to Spirit, by whatever name or in whatever form that Spirit is
recognized. For more information, go to www.lorian.org.

For

Edward
Laurel and Christa

Sorrow looks back
Worry looks around
Faith looks up

Words found on a slip of paper in Ed's pocket.

Table of Contents

Foreword

Claire asked me to provide a foreword and context to her manuscript as a fellow traveler with Parkinson's and I do so with humility. I met Ed and Claire through a mutual friend who introduced us shortly after Ed was diagnosed in 2008. I, myself, was diagnosed in 1992 with symptoms that had revealed themselves 3 or 4 years earlier.

I had been living with PD for close to 20 years when we met and was committed to sharing my experience with others no matter where they were in their disease history. I would often meet with people diagnosed with PD and discuss their questions, fears and concerns while offering some degree of hope that one can live with PD. It is always important to emphasize that everyone's PD is different, each person's path is unique. This book is an expression of the unique path that Ed and Claire took with grace and awareness.

Over the years I explored a variety of avenues of healing and dealing with the many symptoms presented by PD, from herbal medicines to spiritual healers to Deep Brain Stimulation surgery (DBS) to riding a bicycle 2000 miles per year. When presented with decisions about treatment or how best to live with PD, I have found myself seeking inner guidance, trying to hear and listen to a deep sense within myself of what would be best. This was particularly important when it came to deciding about DBS, which was around the time when it was first approved. I was fortunate to have a very successful outcome, which alleviated many of my symptoms, making it possible for me to continue working much longer than I otherwise would have.

Ed and I shared an interest and careers in education leadership and administration, although in quite different settings. His was, at the time I met him, in the founding and leading of a public charter school in western Massachusetts; mine was in the establishment of refugee training programs in Southeast Asia. Our shared careers in education made us questioners.

Ed was intrigued by PD and went beyond the usual questions of possible physical and environmental causes, to more personal and spiritual causes. He had a curiosity about this part of his destiny and what there was to learn on an inner level from this unrelenting disease. Ed and I would meet once a month or so to delve into this topic, in addition to the usual talk of medicines and symptoms. Ed did not shy away from the spiritual questions. He in fact pursued them. As you will see in this account, he and Claire shared a commitment to reflecting together on the spiritual dimensions of living with PD.

At a point when Ed's symptoms were pretty well controlled, he said to another PD person I had introduced him to that he thought PD could be considered a gift. To which that person's wife quickly retorted, "You are early on your path!" Hints of what was to come began to seep into Ed's consciousness. As you will see, Claire shares the harsh reality of what it means to live with a progressive degenerative disease, day after day, both for the person with PD and the caregiver spouse. Ed and I often discussed how our own meetings were a rare opportunity for exploring questions about the spirit within the daily grind, as well as what might be beyond PD in this lifetime, and beyond the veil.

I believe a pivotal point in the disease comes when one can no longer maintain one's own spiritual consciousness. Claire describes this point in Ed's journey, for him, for her, and for their relationship. Ed loses his spiritual anchor in this life and begins living in two worlds. In this world Claire sees him deteriorating into a person she no longer knows. In the other, she feels a deep connection, as evidenced by the synchronicities she cites as confirming indicators of the spiritual world and their shared bond. This is what is beyond PD. A last PD challenge is living through this confusion.

Everyone's PD path is a unique journey to the moments before passing. These moments are almost always shared with others, especially caretakers, family and dear friends. Here one may find oneself asking the same question Ed faced throughout his life on this planet: "What happens when I can no longer be conscious, but my body and altered mind live on?" This book brings the reader through Ed and Claire's journey to the edge of life, beyond Parkinson's Disease.

Spring, 2021
Claude Pepin

Part One

Ed's and my life began to unravel in the fall of 2019. This writing is an attempt to show what the medical experts don't tell you about late stage Parkinson's with dementia. Perhaps they aren't aware that an inner unraveling, as well as the obvious outer unraveling, occurs because their focus is on the outer physical symptoms and the need to provide *something* of a road map, *some* hope for an easy or easier way onwards despite the worsening symptoms. As Ed's neurologist said—more or less—the next to last time we saw him:

"Let's try the higher dosage at 3:00 pm, the lower one in the evening to counter the "off" time in the afternoon..."

"Maybe three sessions of physical therapy a week, not one, would make a difference..."

"If it's helping, the walker is a BIG clue."

Yes, the walker was a BIG clue. Ed had resisted using one for about a year even as, before that, he had resisted using a cane. For him cane and walker were an outright admission he could no longer walk on his own. Even though he was obviously having difficulty walking, the larger difficulty for him for some time was being seen with these aids. Pride can sure be a hard task master!

When I brought the walker home one afternoon, on loan from a friend, Ed circled round it in the back hallway like a sniffing, bristling dog. He folded the folding seat up, tried the hand brakes, squeezed the tires, shrugged, and went back to his office. I parked it in the guest room out of the way of hallway traffic.

Three days later, without telling me what he was up to, Ed took off with it. Upstairs I happened to look out the window of my study, and there was Ed pushing the walker briskly up the road. Very briskly! As had happened now and then, out of the blue, during the previous five years, Ed was suddenly back into upright walking! And he'd barely made it from the kitchen to his office after breakfast, had really been lurching around.

I ran out to join him. But on the way back, the stumbling gait kicked in again, and when we were back in the house he sank down exhausted on the sofa.

I was astonished by this brief sprint, this exhilarating burst of normality. It might have made sense to an observer; an assistive device was assisting a person to walk, as it is designed to do. But the change was so extreme, so dramatic, I was certain something more than that was going on. Was Ed experiencing *kinesia paradoxa*? This is a phenomenon our friend Rob had alerted us to when individuals who typically experience severe difficulties with simple movements may suddenly and briefly perform complex movements quite easily. I thought so and was fascinated by what I saw as the subtle connection between Ed's will to live as he wanted to live and his ability to keep moving. Retrieving, renewing, reversing, healing, white magic: I was open to them all! And I still am.

The walker had triggered something in Ed, in the same way that, for several years before then, a few firm words from the therapist or from me, such as, "Okay, now…. BIG step!" or "MARCH!" said forcefully had called out normal movements. But the walker, like the formerly spoken commands which were no longer effective, not only helped *make* Ed want to walk, the walker also made the unraveling evident. The unraveling not only of fluid forward movement but of Ed's pride.

Then, right then, the unraveling of other things also could be sensed, the most difficult of which, for me, were the threads that had bound us together for over 50 years. It is primarily the unraveling of our relationship that I want to share here, not so much as a warning to other couples where one spouse may be entering the late stage of PD (I will use this abbreviation for Parkinson's from here on) without any sense of how hard it can be, but as a challenge to stay open, open to other ways of discovering connection, relationship and love when body and brain are obviously faltering, failing, stopping.

Ed passed over April 19, 2020

At Thanksgiving of 2019 our family noticed what I'd been living with daily—and sometimes crying about without knowing

2

exactly what I was crying about—the rapid worsening of the PD symptoms.

Ed and I thought maybe the worsening symptoms had to do with the medications wearing off faster or boomeranging back on him, knocking him off balance. We spent quite a bit of time keeping track of his daily intake of these medications and their effect on him, especially in association with what and when he ate, as it's said the digestive system can interfere with the effect of carbidopa-levodopa (which was then Ed's primary medication.)

Ed also felt new dread at the possibility of worsening cognitive decline. He was aware he was losing many things: eyeglasses, cell phone, car keys, wallet, checkbook, his canes, jackets, sweaters, even shoes, and forgetting names, schedules, appointments, even how to get to appointments, and more. In an effort to meet this dread headlong, Ed decided to exercise his brain by memorizing a poem. The one he picked was a poem we first read together shortly after we met, *God's Grandeur* by Gerard Manley Hopkins. A magnificent but hard to memorize hymn to the Divine:

> The world is charged with the grandeur of God.
> It will flame out, like shining from shook foil;
> It gathers to a greatness, like the ooze of oil
> Crushed. Why do men then now not reck his rod?
> Generations have trod, have trod, have trod;
> And all is seared with trade; bleared, smeared with toil;
> And wears man's smudge and shares man's smell: the soil
> Is bare now, nor can foot feel, being shod.
>
> And for all this, nature is never spent;
> There lives the dearest freshness deep down things;
> And though the last lights off the black West went
> Oh, morning, at the brown brink eastward, springs—
> Because the Holy Ghost over the bent
> World broods with warm breast and with ah! bright wing.

A month later, at Christmas, the family was, again, startled by the rapidly worsening PD. And I was still having crying spells when driving home after swimming at the YMCA, without knowing exactly what I was crying about.

Without turning this into an autobiography, I want to speak about Ed's and my relationship because everything that happened later, especially during his last three months, was shaped by that.

At this point we'd known one another 53 years and had been married almost 52 years. I'm profoundly deaf, since having mumps at the age of six. Ed was the kindest man I'd ever met when we met at age 22. At the heart of this kindness was the fact that my deafness was never a limiting factor in the relationship. Without any fanfare or fuss, Ed helped me find my home in the hearing world. He knew me as a person rather than primarily as a deaf person. Sure, I needed to read his lips and would look to him for help making phone calls, following conversations in large gatherings, understanding speakers in conferences or making sense of sounds I heard through my hearing aid, and later, through my cochlear implant. He'd fill me in on radio programs and, before closed captioning was available, TV and films. And I, in turn, would share with him whatever I heard or saw between the lines of what was being said. This—the unspoken things people often convey—which can be at odds with the words coming out of their mouths—was a source of discovery, amazement and humor for both of us.

Ed and I developed our own language of facial expressions, gestures, movements and touch. I'm sure, even without deafness being a part of the picture, this happens to all couples. We were so attuned, we often thought of the same thing at the same moment and regularly finished each other's sentences. When Ed was diagnosed with PD, I could sense the effects of the symptoms without his having to describe them in detail, if at all. It was possible to see, for example, by the stoop of his shoulders, when the freezing of gait was coming on. Or, his fatigue could be so oppressive, I'd feel it as a heaviness in the atmosphere when I stepped into his study. Likewise, the look on his face when he woke in the morning said volumes. Sometimes he'd be listening to the news, eager to sound off on the most recent political atrocities. Other times it was extremely hard for him to be back in his body. Simply lifting or swinging his legs to the side of the bed to sit up appeared to be a Herculean task.

4

When the unraveling of which I am speaking began, our private language was affected, which was rattling to both of us. Physical challenges we could figure out together, but these psychological challenges were like Hydras. No sooner did I think we'd put one misinterpretation to rest than two more would pop up. Ed often thought I hadn't heard him and would accuse me of bluffing when in fact we were no longer in the same place within a conversation.

Should I point this out to Ed? Should I say, "I told you about this an hour ago" which he might hear as an accusation, or should I just let it pass? Honesty had always been a cornerstone of our relationship and suddenly the question became, 'IS honesty the kindest way to be with the kind man I married?" That similar misinterpretations and misunderstandings were happening to Ed with others also was, I'll admit, a relief to me.

Ed's confusions and cognitive decline made me aware of two other things. First, we hadn't, when in conversation together over the years, only connected through thoughts in our brains, but though thoughts in our hearts. We both knew when we were having inspired and inspiring conversations and would emerge from them feeling in complete agreement not only with each other but with something larger. I've experienced this with other people also, not just with Ed, but, with Ed, conversations of this sort usually had to do with the direction our life was taking. Now as the sense of mutual togetherness and agreement began to fray, the sense of a direction began to disappear. In the earlier stages of PD there had been occasions when I didn't know where Ed was—and he didn't know where he was either—but he was able to acknowledge and discuss his own puzzlement, so we'd be back together again. But now he was, more and more, definitely elsewhere.

The second thing I became aware of was that, despite this unraveling and loss of direction, the keystone of our life together *was* still there. The keystone was the promise we had agreed on to *"protect, border and salute"* one another in this life-time. Those italicized words, from Rainer Maria Rilke (in *Letters to a Young Poet*) were woven into the vow we composed and said to each other when we created our marriage ceremony.

This may all sound quite lofty; we certainly weren't fully

conscious of what we were saying when we said that vow, yet the blessings of the union held us to it. And most of the time what we were holding to had nothing to do with great revelations or great temptations—had, quite simply, to do with mundane everyday things: Who was going to comfort the crying baby at 2 :00 am? Would Ed tire of being my interpreter? How often would I have to put up with Ed working overtime? (Which he had done pretty consistently even in earlier years when the family was packed and waiting by the car to go on vacation. Later, it dawned on me this may have been an early manifestation of PD.)

Our relationship worked its way pretty seamlessly through the various challenges, because we usually responded in a similar manner, with a sense of humor and plenty of hugs. But, most importantly, each took to heart the deepest needs, hopes and dreams of the other. There were times when my aspirations were more important to Ed than his own, and vice versa. He was always fully committed to his work in education, wherever he was employed, and I always knew I had to write. Each of our work "callings" demanded some self-sacrifice of the other, and that we both did gladly, without any hesitation.

But PD wasn't a work or calling either of us had asked for though we did make a big effort to meet it as an opportunity. An opportunity to learn about the human body and brain and the marvels of conscious and beautiful movement. An opportunity to learn about boundaries, patience, resilience, and true friendship, not just with each other but with quite a few others. Above all, an opportunity to go *into* prayer.

And PD demanded a degree of self-sacrifice I'd never known existed. For Ed this sacrifice is best described as "an erasure of self" –a term someone with PD (I don't know who) coined. Bit by bit, year by year, then faster and faster at the end, the PD hacked away at Ed's ability to move, use his hands, be expressive, speak, respond, reach out and relate to others, care for himself, think, remember...

This erasure of self was very definitely behind the unraveling of our relationship. First the PD hacked away at the things we wanted to do, both together and on our own, then the things we'd been able to do together, then the things we never thought we'd have to do together. All of these losses had us reeling as I'll show in some of the incidents I want to share from Ed's last month and a half. But when we reached the point when it was clear, I myself could no longer do everything for Ed, and that, in turn, led to our physical separation which was enforced by the lockdown on account of COVID, *then* I again found the keystone of this life we had chosen to live together. The vow we'd made to each other then was coming back, and it was asking for something new and different from both of us.

Part Two

Almost every morning during the twelve years after Ed was diagnosed with PD, we sat together for half an hour, more or less, to read and pray. We read in quite a few books, among them *How to Know Higher Worlds* by Rudolf Steiner, *Open Mind Open Heart* by Thomas Keating and several of David Spangler's books on what he calls Incarnational Spirituality. Again and again our readings helped calm, guide, inspire and fortify us.

Just before Ed's first hospitalization, we started reading a book by our friend Thomas Yeomans , *Holy Fire : The Process of Soul Awakening*. The other morning, when I dipped into *Holy Fire* again after a long break from it, I opened *exactly* to the pages Ed and I had read together before he left home and found myself back in that cold, grey Saturday morn. And I was astonished by how right-on the words felt. I believe the two quotes that follow helped ease the acute anxiety around the validity of his consciousness that Ed was subject to as the PD worsened. I believe they reassured him, the very essence of him, that his soul, was intact—always—even as everything was unraveling and we were being forced apart.

I (Tom is speaking) have come to use the word "soul" to express the experience of the core of consciousness in each of us that holds the potential and pattern of our full, unique maturity. This soul is seeking realization and expression in our everyday life and its presence is within us from birth to death. (p.32)

And a bit further on:

Our consciousness is at the core of the soul journey, but the journey proceeds even if we do not pay conscious attention to it. We grow up the best we can, even if we are quite unconscious of how this is happening, and the soul journey in this sense does not depend on our being aware of it. **Life seeks to live itself more deeply regardless.** (p.34 I've put the last line in bold.)

During the morning time, Ed and I often discussed things on our minds and also, as I mentioned above, said prayers for others, our country, the world, the earth and those who had passed over. Occasionally we found ourselves asking what we meant by "prayer," particularly when people asked us to pray for them. Were we sending prayers or blessings? One, the other, or both? What's the difference between the two? Can we actually send *something*? If so, exactly *what*? And what if someone doesn't want that something? In the past, Ed had had moments when he'd been annoyed when others told him they were praying for him. As we pondered these matters, I believe we may have been, quite unconsciously, testing the strength of our personal interweavings, as well as those with others. Like checking out the condition of the ropes before going to sea. I'll come back to this later, when Ed and I were no longer able to be together, and I found myself praying for, and with, him.

We usually observed this time around 8:30 or 9 :00 am, but then Ed began sleeping later and later and taking longer and longer to get up. He had to take his first round of medications at 7 :00 am — I'd help him sit up to swallow them — but started falling asleep again after that. By the time he was actually up, had had breakfast and was thinking about getting dressed, we were well into the day, the next round of medications had to be taken, the phone was often ringing, we had appointments to get to, and so on. Ed periodically resolved to get going earlier but couldn't hold to the resolve for long, and I didn't want to become a nag. A brief, "better-something-than-nothing" sit down time around 11:00 am often ensued.

How could it be that a retired couple suddenly didn't have time to be together? Yes, of course, we were together, day after day, yet the central focus of that together time was the PD and how to manage, ease, outwit, forget, or simply endure it. I believe in being willing to let go of patterns that are no longer helpful, but neither of us was ready to give up the morning time outright. So, to counter the trend that was working its way into our morning anchoring time, we tried a different observance. Before saying grace at dinner, we'd take turns sharing a special experience from the day. That made us *look* for things to share. Things like the chipmunk that was trying hard and persistently to slip through the door when I brought the groceries in, or a vivid dream from the night before, or a story Ed had heard on the radio. But this didn't last long, because we often ate when the News Hour was starting, and both of us couldn't help but be interested in the political dramas playing out; those *were* pretty effective distractions from the PD! Also, as I came to realize, Ed not only didn't feel he had anything to share by 6 :00 pm — late afternoons and early evenings being major low-tide times for him — he didn't like feeling obliged to share.

We then hit on the idea of introducing something entirely different at dessert time, Mad-Libs or a simple game, or getting to know an artist, writer or poet one of us liked and admired. I quickly zeroed in on the writing of Brian Doyle whom I'd discovered a few years earlier. Ed never said no when I asked him if him if he wanted "a Brian Doyle" anytime of the day, not just with dessert. That usually meant a "proem" (prose-poem) from *A Shimmer of Something : Lean Stories of Spiritual Substance*. Doyle's writing is good with anything: ice cream, burnt toast, the damn medications.

Brian Doyle's life-affirming writing nourished us — me particularly — as our life together continued to unravel, less praying together, less talking together (more staring at TV together) less sharing of what we were doing. Ed was working less and less on the lathe (it was, in fact, becoming dangerous), I couldn't settle into my pastels, and Ed, who'd always been my first and most helpful critic, became indifferent to the pages I left on his desk. If I asked if he had read them, he often couldn't find them. Our girls were wonderful about reaching out to him regularly by phone; Laurel called him *every* week, and I know how much he appreciated that. Yet, when Christa mentioned in passing how her father no longer asked her during their conversations about her work, on the phone or in person, I felt with a shock, "Yup! It's that way for me too."

Then knew with a sharp pang, "Hey, wait! This **isn't** him…. he's being taken from us."

During one of our rare morning times at the start of January, when we were able to sit down together before 11:00 am, Ed remembered a day, a week earlier, when he woke and "felt okay." Gladdened by his willingness to converse, I asked if he meant okay physically. Was he expressing longing for some of the better days or was he expressing fleeting release from frustration with the freezing of gait, difficulty getting up, occasional difficulty swallowing, constipation et cetera?

Ed paused, as though feeling his way around his body, then feeling his way around his soul, then said very quietly while looking out the window that he was okay with where he was in life, with the life he'd lived, and with having to die.

Tears instantly formed in my eyes blurring my vision. I'd been having more and more moments when I knew his departure was coming. During one of them, maybe nine months before then, I *knew* he wasn't going to live to be 80. Making it to 80 had been his wish on his 64th birthday, the day he received the PD diagnosis. I didn't share that intuition with him, that knowing that felt as obvious as the sun sinking out of sight at the end of the day. I simply pushed it away.

After recollecting his okay moment, Ed turned to me, saw my tears and added quite forcefully, "**Not yet!**"

What he meant was, "Yes, I'm ready, but, **NO,** not now!"

I believe Ed was acknowledging the unraveling and trying somehow to halt it. Neither of us said anything more, we were like two scared kids.

Ed became obsessed towards the end of January with cleaning his office. He made piles of files and notebooks on the floor and directed Anne to carry them downstairs. We had found and hired Anne, who was in her mid 60s, to be his companion for two hours a week. The thinking was that I'd get to swim my laps at the YMCA and wouldn't have to drive him both to and from physical therapy that day, and Ed would get fun time with someone new. I felt badly for Anne, though. She'd been enthusiastic about the prospect of taking him out to lunch after PT or to museums or art shows, and here was Ed literally ordering her to carry heavy boxes wherever he happened to think they should go. He also went well over Anne's two hours one day when he decided he needed to go to the shopping mall forty-five minutes away to purchase another vacuum cleaner for me. I was moved by the thought that he wanted to lighten my load any way he could, even if we didn't need a new vacuum. (Ed also asked Anne to help him get a birthday gift for me: enough wild bird seed to last about two years! Unfortunately, first mice, then a bear, got wind of that birthday gift in the garage. Whatever I could salvage did go to the birds.)

As Ed's clean-up efforts expanded and intensified, new piles of messes appeared not only in his wood shop, in the garage, on his side of the bedroom, but also in his office, the place he was determined to unclutter. There were broken flashlights, lamp shades, radios and clocks all over his desktop. Anne and I discovered duplicate bags of replacement parts he must have purchased when still able to drive.

Then there were the piles of shoes, boots and slippers on the floor beside his desk. Several times when I brought Ed his late morning or early afternoon medications and a glass of water, I found him wearing a single sock and shoe on one foot. At first, I was amused and reminded him of lines he'd chanted from *Mother Goose* when our girls were toddlers:

Diddle Diddle Dumpling, my son John (or my daughter Laurel)
One shoe off and one shoe on...

Then, the second or third time that happened, it hit me: he wasn't paying attention to what he was doing. It looked as though he'd started putting his socks and shoes on and, half -way through, was distracted by something else, so went off to that, forgetting about the sock and shoe for the bare foot. It *was* difficult getting his socks and shoes on; no wonder his attention wandered. His legs and feet were very swollen. I had to help him often with my fingers or the shoehorn. Boots particularly could become lumpy, cumbersome, claustrophobic objects.

It sometimes felt during these moments as though Ed's ongoing struggle with socks and shoes, and later, briefly, with pants, wasn't merely another angle on the festination and freezing up. Meaning, if shoes, socks and pants, made it that much harder to walk, to heck with them! The struggle had spread from walking normally, to standing up straight, to keeping his balance, to getting his clothing, socks and shoes on for being upright. It felt as though Ed was beginning to want OUT! Out of all these tiresome routines and obstacle courses, out of the endless fatigue, out of his leaden, clumsy body.

The wisdom in Ed's hands was also unraveling, which, for me, was more distressing than the unraveling of his walking abilities. When I speak of the "wisdom" of Ed's hands unraveling, I'm not referring to the PD tremor, which he'd had in his right hand and down his right side when first diagnosed but which had pretty much disappeared by this time and had been replaced by other PD symptoms. For me, the sense of balance, the sense of touch, and the sense of speech comprise this wisdom. (I know there are likely more such inherent abilities or powers to the hands than I'm naming here.)

Even if armed with canes, ski poles, the walker or hand grips, Ed began to experience difficulty at this time staying upright. Several times when standing, his hands would suddenly fly out as if reaching for a wall that wasn't there. A few times he fell over and narrowly missed hitting his head on the furniture or the floor. When sitting beside him on the sofa or lying beside him in bed I realized he was off-balance and off-touch as to the placement of his body in the space we were sharing. When it began, I teased him about pushing me off the sofa and out of bed, but when it continued and I knew he wasn't teasing me back, I started thinking about getting a bed rail.

Ed was depending more and more on my assistance with dressing, undressing, buttoning, zipping, tying, cutting, typing, turning pages, combing his hair, opening doors… everything! There were frequent accidents: plates and glasses getting broken, food falling, the computer or his cell phone malfunctioning because he couldn't find or hit the right keys. It was humiliating. His hands were no longer the hands I'd known so well: carving, sanding, painting, hammering, switching light bulbs, hauling storm windows up the ladder and fastening them to the house with the power screwdriver, opening jars I couldn't open, paddling the canoe, washing dishes, squeezing my shoulders, reaching for my hand in the dark. That Ed clearly felt helpless in the presence of his more and more helpless hands made me also feel helpless.

That our hands possess a sense of speech—or language—requires some explanation.

To go back a step, briefly: the face, of course, speaks, is always speaking even when one isn't using words to talk. And, as anyone related to a person with PD knows, the PD mask can greatly diminish and dull the language of the face. I noticed soon after Ed was first diagnosed how people would talk more to me than to him and knew it was because they couldn't read his face. The mask was hiding him, he wasn't hiding behind it. Without being aware of it, they couldn't find the common facial responses we exchange with others when conversing. They didn't know how to tell if he was listening, not-listening, was tired or bored, and so turned, instead, to me. Ed's PD mask was hard for me, as a face and lip reader, but, fortunately, it was confined to the lower part of his face. I could find him in his eyes, though his eyes too were sometimes weary, veiled, and later, briefly, darkened.

The PD mask made the language of Ed's arms and hands all the more important and he knew this. He tried to be more present, less aloof, when greeting people, tried to be more expansive in his appreciation of others. He kept finding new and funnier ways of speaking through the movements of his hands and arms during the five years we were in our PD Dance class. Dancing, mirroring, improvising all became ways of pushing back against the constrictive, silencing, muting forces of PD.

Just when the PD was starting to clamp down yet harder on Ed's movements I heard of the PD Pantomime Project, and its founder, Rob Mermin (who is mentioned earlier in connection with *kinesia paradoxa*) came to give a workshop in our area. For me Rob's workshop, what he shared of his own fully conscious way of meeting PD rather than letting oneself be pulled into its undertow, the gentle always respectful way he moves with and through space, and the presence of his teacher and mentor Marcel Marceau in his work, was an enormous help, a real tonic. Through Marcel Marceau and Rob, I began to see and understand how our first language *is* movement and our hands and arms particularly, as the energy in them radiates out from our hearts (or are closed to that energy — for our hands and arms *can* close to it) are in constant dialogue with the world. This seeing stays with me and, although it was not of special significance to Ed in his last

15

two months because of the rapid unraveling of his whole life, it was of help later as he was passing over. And it remains very much on my radar, as something I know is important and believe needs to be better understood and worked with on many levels.

It was Sunday evening. A couple we'd known for almost as long as we'd been married had been with us for the weekend and had just departed. Ed and I both knew, from their faces, how shocked they were by Ed's condition. We tried, in our different ways, to reassure them we were the exact same people, things weren't as bad as they looked—or were they? Their car wasn't even out of sight when I said to Ed, "Does it have to be this exhausting to be with dear, old friends?" He felt the same. The weekend hadn't only exhausted him, it had depressed him.

I was in my study responding to emails when I heard him calling for help. I raced downstairs and found him bent over the kitchen sink. From the way Ed was holding his left hand with his right hand, my first thought was he'd broken something. Then I saw he was holding his ring finger which was bent and swollen. He'd had unsuccessful surgery on the middle muscles of that hand 6 years earlier to reposition them as they'd been damaged when he played football as a teen. It would've helped a lot if that operation had been done when he was a teen, but it hadn't, and now the hand was becoming more and more bent and arthritic making it harder and harder for him to do any woodworking.

Ed said the wedding band *had* to come off, it was too tight. I remembered the story of my grandpa waking in the middle of the night because his wedding band was affecting the circulation in his hand. He ran out to the woodshed in his nightshirt and cap and cut the band off with metal shears. Grandpa running around in his nightshirt and cap? It became a family joke. It was a joke too that Grandma and Grandpa had always been a tad cantankerous with one another, even the youngest of us knew that.

But this was no joking matter; Ed's hand was swelling. I lathered it up with warm water and soap and pulled at the ring. No luck. I next tried using a soapy ribbed washcloth to get a better grip. Again, no luck. I couldn't get it over the knuckle which now looked like an enormous fat walnut.

I suggested getting metal shears from Ed's wood shop but he didn't want it cut. Nor did he want to go to the ER.

Ed said *he* would pull it off, *had* to pull it off, and for me to pour liquid dish detergent over that hand as he pulled. I got the jumbled feeling that he couldn't find the words to express the urgency he felt right then. And this urgency had to do with releasing me from having to care for him. He wanted that badly. As if by getting the wedding band off he could release me.

Ed almost yelled at me to get going pouring the detergent. I was so startled I squeezed the bottle of detergent as hard as I could and was immediately afraid—from the way he was bending over and exerting himself, his left arm flat against the kitchen counter, the hand over the sink—he might break part of his hand.

Then suddenly—the ring was off!

I dropped the bottle of detergent and grabbed him before he toppled over.

No broken bones, thank goodness!

I wrapped his left hand in an ice pack. The next day I saw that, not only had his hand turned black and blue, his whole arm was bruised. And it remained bruised for over a week. Fritha, our PD dance class instructor, was aware something was off with Ed's left arm, even though he always wore a long-sleeved shirt. Inquired, took a look, and was sobered by what she found.

When the ring came off I jokingly said, "Now, you're free!" (I had made his ring and he had made mine. His was quite a bit thicker than mine and, though round, you could see when it was held up how two interwoven gold wires created a five point star. Mine is much thinner yet also makes a five-point star when held up.)

Ed wasn't in a joking mood; he didn't even smile.

He left his wedding band, forgotten, on the windowsill over the kitchen sink. It stayed there for about a week. Later when I put it in my jewelry box, Ed didn't notice it had been moved.

(Equally strange was how, later on, Ed's wedding ring disappeared. About a week after he died, I took his band out of my jewelry box and put it on my right ring finger—opposite the thin band on my left hand. A few hours later when Face Timing with

Christa, I noticed the ring finger on my right hand was bare. I hadn't realized Ed's ring was so loose, it had slipped right off! I looked and looked for it—unsuccessfully. The entire family has also looked for it—unsuccessfully. As I didn't leave the house that day, beyond walking to our mailbox, I believe it will reappear at some point.)

We began sleeping apart. Ed needed to get up frequently at night to relieve himself (we had, some years before, figured out a way for him to do that without his having to walk to the bathroom) and this put me on "high alert." It seemed as though he'd no sooner gotten up once than he needed to get up again. He could also be wide awake during these times and that had me concerned he was becoming a "sundowner." (A condition in the elderly associated with impaired cognition and sleep rhythms. A sun downer might wake thinking 3:00 am is 3:00 pm.)

Sensing this was rather stressful for me, Ed decided to sleep in his sleeping bag on the small foldout sofa in his office, and we followed a different bedtime routine for about two weeks. After helping him into his night clothes, I'd zip him up in his sleeping bag, everything he thought he might need – cane, flashlight, graham crackers, water and the remote control for the TV within easy reach—then would sing, as with the Mother Goose, one or two of the lullabies we'd sung to our daughters when they were infants. There was also a finger-play song around closing the eyes (drawing the eyelids down over the eyes), closing the shutters (turning the ear flaps inwards towards the eyes), closing the door (gently pinching the mouth shut) then turning the key (making a turning motion on the lips). It was all meant lightly, playfully, but Ed was totally present, altogether serious, every time we did this routine. A bit *too* serious. There was something dark in his eyes that I hadn't seen before, it was almost spooky. I stopped the singing, and Ed abruptly announced he was moving back upstairs.

As Ed's nighttime waking continued, I'd often move downstairs to finish the night on the sofa. I'd lie there in the dark, looking out the window at the stars, sensing their timelessness, agelessness, perpetuity. They made the night air more breathable, gave me renewed feelings of space extending out and out, and, amazingly, order in that infinite space. Most importantly, the stars gave me a needed feeling of independence. When I woke in the morning after being with the stars in this way, there was more space *in* me, space and also strength to go on.

I have a vivid memory of our last visit to Ed's neurologist, Dr. G. We had an appointment for February 11th (our appointments with him were three or more months apart the drive to his office a bit over two hours), but I felt dizzy and nauseous that day. It was the first time we had ever canceled, and I felt guilty because I'd been emailing regularly with Dr. G about Ed's worsening PD symptoms and possible changes in the medications. Ed and I both had been wanting urgently to confer in person with him. Ed wanted to hear why he had not been accepted into the clinical trial Dr. G had encouraged us months before to apply to. We had applied, and I know Ed pinned a lot of hope on that trial despite the crazy amount of driving being in it would have entailed.

About five hours after we bowed out of the February 11th appointment, the secretary in the scheduling department informed us the next available time with Dr. G was in July. That made me feel even worse.

However, a week later when a friend was at our house helping us sort through a maze of insurance phone calls, the phone rang. Dr. G's office was calling to let us know there was an opening that very day, in three hours, at 3:30 pm. Did we want it? Yes! I, for one, sure did! Ed and I were in the car within half an hour and on our way.

I used the special parking permit to park quite close to the hospital entrance, yet still there was the walk slightly uphill. Ed was pushing the walker up the incline and I was helping him, holding one side of the walker, keeping it steady so he wouldn't veer off the sidewalk. The doorman ran down to assist us, saying Ed really needed a wheelchair. The man was shocked, as though unsure I realized how poorly Ed looked. Another doorman then appeared with a wheelchair which Ed sank into.

I wheeled Ed to the neurology department, we checked in, then had to wait an hour before we were called. That annoyed Ed no end. He wasn't his usual charming self when the nurse took his blood pressure and weight. After that, she put us in the room beside Dr.

G's office, rather than having us return to the waiting room.

About twenty minutes later a couple, maybe five or six years younger than us, emerged from the doctor's office. As the door was wide open, we could see what a spirited exchange they were having with Dr. G. There was much laughter. It was clear, from his posture, that the gentleman had PD and his stride was, still, pretty good. And the wife — there was no question she was his wife — was holding their parkas, her pocketbook, a canvas bag very much like Ed's, and the papers Dr. G usually handed the caregiver. I remember thinking, "Golly, they're us when we first met Dr. G." I'd never thought before how we probably look like a certain type. An older, greying, Land's End or LL Bean couple!

Then the bright smile on Dr. G's face dimmed when he caught sight of Ed. I knew he was seeing what he hadn't seen three and a half months earlier: the unraveling.

Dear Ed rose — as he always had — to greet Dr. G. I don't just mean physically. As he stood up, Ed rose in mood to meet his PD doctor. He was remarkable the way he stepped into his gracious self, in spirit, and as well as he could in body. He was actually — even before we entered Dr. G's office — a bit feisty and confrontational as to why he hadn't been admitted to the clinical trial.

Dr. G, a little taken back by Ed's question, offered us chairs and explained again, as he had online, that only one person had been picked from his pool of three or four possible PD candidates.

Ed said he thought his cognitive decline was behind his rejection in this trial. Right then there was no beating around the bush with him. It was as though he, Ed, was making the diagnosis. He haltingly described forgetting things, not being able to find the words he wanted to say what he wanted, not being able to type or, if he did type, not being able to remember how to get into emails or the patient portal, and so on.

I noticed that Ed did not mention the "worms" he'd been seeing for several months — tiny, white worms here and there on the sofa, rug, towels, his clothing, or in his hair. I'd decided while driving I would bring the worms up later in connection with the medications. (Christa had emailed me online PD information on this very topic, in connection with warnings about the meds.) Ed truly believed he was seeing worms, live worms. He even tried catching them in jars and would point out bits of dust in these jars as proof he'd caught and killed these worms. It might have been denial on my part, yet Ed's fixation on "cognitive decline" and the fact that he was truly upset by what he was forgetting and could flare up more and more unexpectedly when I pointed out he'd forgotten, made me very wary of bringing up the topic of hallucinations. Cognitive decline was enough hallucinations was a whole other topic.

I saw, too, how intently Dr. G was listening to Ed, how his listening eyes moved back and forth between us during that appointment and felt, in a sad, sinking way, "This good man is coming to the end of the help he can offer us."

Having expressed his anxiety around cognitive decline, Ed eased back into his usual quieter, more reflective, way of being, while I gave Dr. G the usual summary I'd typed up for the February 11th appointment we had missed. The summary of the medication schedule we'd been following and how things had been going since we'd last been with him.

He glanced over it quickly. I knew it sounded like all the previous summaries. The same points of concern, the same complaints and questions had been coming up for months, and I knew, from Dr. G's face, I was hammering it home, as usual: What-can-we-do? *Please-*what-can-we-do? **HELP**-what-can-we-do?

That summary brought us all back to the fact that our time with the doctor was monitored, appointments are limited and expensive, that Dr. G was in demand and there aren't enough neurologists for the many folks being diagnosed with PD. Dr. G then switched from being engaged listener to efficient scientist-doctor at the computer playing with possible tricks he might be able to conjure up by switching doses around or trying other meds. He did suggest another possible medication and gave us a glossy promotional flyer about it to read at home. This other med—it was almost like he was suggesting a vacation to some place we'd never dreamt of going—might be able to address the "cognitive decline" issues. I noticed how the couple on the cover of the flyer he handed us were handsome, healthy looking, holding hands.

The sense of it turning into a "regular" appointment made Ed

21

perk up. Maybe he hadn't made it into the clinical trial, but perhaps there would be another. We became chatty like the couple that had been there before us. Would Dr. G himself ever do a clinical trial like the one he'd suggested when we first met him of getting PD patients into fly fishing? Dr.G's smile returned. Hope was in the air again.

To my amazement—and Dr. G's too—when we all stood to say good-bye, Ed grabbed the handles on the wheelchair and pushed it out and down the hall!

Dr. G and I exchanged a quick, astonished look and hurried after Ed. What had become of the man who couldn't make it to the front entrance with the walker? Was I again witnessing *kinesia paradoxa*?

However, as soon as we were back in the lobby, the freezing returned full force and Ed sank back into the wheelchair, almost missing the seat as I helped him down.

When we got to where the walker had been left and Ed was, again, behind it and back in his parka, it felt too risky for him to go down the hill to where the car was parked. I told Ed to wait right outside the main entrance and explained I'd drive the car up to fetch him.

There were no doormen on duty this time, and when I returned with the car there was no sign of Ed either outside or just inside. I asked a bearded guy waiting near the entrance if he'd seen a man with a walker walking off, and he shook his head.

I parked the car by the curb, put on the emergency lights and dashed inside to find him. No sign anywhere in the lobby of Ed. Panic rose up: had I lost my husband?

I glanced outside again, then back into the lobby, and there— stumbling out of the men's room in a daze—was Ed!

I ran over to him and he yelled, "WHY DID YOU LEAVE ME?"

"I've been looking for you," I said quietly. "I thought I was going to pick you up by the front door, the car's out there."

"BUT YOU LEFT ME!" He was furious. His eyes were not the steady brown eyes I'd always known.

"Come...." I took his arm. "Let's get you into the car."

Then I looked around, "Where's the walker?" We needed it badly to get him to the car.

Luckily a man who was nearby and had overheard our exchange,

22

stepped into the men's room and appeared a second later with the walker.

Ed latched onto it and we made our way out to the car. He was still muttering about my deserting him.

"Cognitive decline" right then, firmly and truly became the bottom line on that last visit to Dr. G.

In the fall I had gotten the impression "cognitive decline" was one thing, hallucinations were another. I did mention the worm hallucinations briefly to Dr. G in the visit just described but we didn't discuss them in person. I didn't, right then, want Ed to feel I was challenging his accounts of his experience, especially in front of others. As was evident when he thought I'd forgotten him at the hospital, confrontational qualities he'd never exhibited before were emerging. Nor did I email with Dr. G about the worms, for I shared everything I wrote to the doctor and his nurses with Ed as long as we were together in person. This changed overnight when Ed went into the hospital, then the nursing home.

Seeing worms here and there—and I knew they *weren't* worms—seemed minor beside the other challenges, like the continual waking at night. Also, did I *really* know what Ed's mental experiences were like? No, I did not. That I was approaching a point where I couldn't really advocate for Ed, because I couldn't get into his experiences and be with him, was all a part of this unraveling process. And it wasn't merely an unraveling process, it was becoming a parting process.

I need here to go back a step for a few minutes.

There's plenty of talk about cognitive decline today and certainly not only in connection with PD, though it's often referred to in the literature on PD. When I forget something the common joke is I'm having a "senior moment" or am in the early stage of "cognitive decline." As I trust I've made clear, Ed was super sensitive to these trains of thought especially when he knew he was forgetting quite a few small things and getting other, often bigger, things mixed up. (He had at this point, for example, gotten the last names of his daughters and son's-in law mixed up. He unknowingly gave a lawyer the name of his older daughter as being married to the husband of her sister.)

I, too, am sensitive to the warning, or joking, comments on "cognitive decline." My mother died from a series of strokes that rendered her more and more incoherent, and my father had a slowly worsening dementia during his last five years. Ed and I, however, believed we all have a conscious mind, which is part of our soul, as well as a physical brain, and most of the attention in connection with "cognitive decline" is on the physical brain. We never questioned the scientific evidence that PD and dementia (and other conditions, deafness included) affect certain parts of the physical brain. Nor did we doubt the profound assistance medications can bring to these affected or damaged parts of the brain. We experienced firsthand how carbidopa-levodopa gave relief from the PD stiffness and, for some years, helped with the gait difficulties. (Though less, and then less so, as the PD advanced.) Ed was not a good candidate for deep brain stimulation, for reasons I won't go into here, but we were always curious about it and read up on it on behalf of friends who'd had it or were considering having it. We were also very interested in and admiring of the research being done in medicine and physical therapy in connection with the "plasticity" of the brain and ways different parts of the brain can be found to assist or take over functions of the affected parts. Yet we always believed, even before PD, that we are quite a bit more than human beings with physical brains and bodies.

As had happened with my dad as his dementia progressed, I got the impression Ed, though he was forgetting things in the linear everyday world, was not becoming unaware, unintelligent, purposeless. Rather, I felt Ed's awareness shifting to other things. There was the decline of short-term memory and his interest in various "files" in his long-term memory, like stories about early boyhood escapades, girlfriends he'd had whom I'd never met, relatives I hardly knew, various jobs he'd had, and travels he'd taken. There was a fair amount of circling back, a kind of weaving-the-past-into-the-present quality to this, but it seemed to me he was also wakening—or reawakening— to other ways of looking at and into the world. The natural world especially.

In the morning Ed sometimes referred with wonder to the

24

quality of light in our yard and how the wind was talking but he couldn't quite get what it was saying. What he shared was very real and beautiful. He also pointed out to family and friends, various rocks and trees he loved and felt he communed with. He also often with assistance wanted to go to a certain spot by a river where he'd fished. He'd sit there, perched atop a rock, eyes on the flowing water. Likewise, he would lie, when it was warm enough, in a sun chair on our lawn, eyes on the land or the sky. I wanted to ask him *what* he was looking at, *what* he was seeing, but the question felt invasive, so refrained. It was as though he was being called out into the flowing water, into the landscape and the clouds above, in the same way I was being called out by the stars at night. In one way this felt to me like *more* unraveling—Ed going "off" God knows where—yet on a deeper level, and this feeling predominated, I felt I was holding to our marriage vow. In short, I was protecting him as best as I could, and bordering him, in the sense of standing with him, and saluting him in the necessary solitude of his onward journey.

Ed also talked now and then of sensing non-physical beings on the periphery of his vision. We debated who they might be and how he might address and possibly engage with them. The veil between the two worlds was, for him, becoming more transparent and it was important to me that he know this as an opportunity, rather than fearing people, particularly doctors, might view it as feeble-mindedness. We referred to this as his journey into other dimensions of being and forms of consciousness. This was not simply push-back to the times when we got yet another article or email from someone on "cognitive decline" or "Late-Stage PD Dementia," I know this was Ed connecting with deeper places in himself.

To summarize: Ed *was* experiencing "cognitive decline", knew that, and was frustrated and frightened by it. This cognitive decline *was*, as I saw it, connected to his physical brain and very possibly also to the hallucinations he experienced. I think these happenings, considering the onslaught by PD, were inevitable, even as physical decline and death *are* inevitable.

But—and Ed always believed this as I do too--one isn't just a physical body with a physical brain, that may undergo decline and malfunction; one also has a soul and a spirit which are capable of transcendent love and expanding consciousness, both within and outside of the physical body. (I can hardly begin to say how important this belief was and is.)

It felt to me as though Ed's soul and spirit were struggling valiantly to stay interwoven and on course as his physical body unraveled, and he somehow had to experience release from even that effort in order to get to wherever he was going. I could hear this struggle in the experiences he was having and comments he made during the two weeks before he was first hospitalized. Those two weeks were really the last time we had together in person as a married couple.

In the middle of the night of March 1st Ed woke me. He was sitting on the edge of his side of the bed shaking. I turned on the light and grabbed him from behind by the shoulders, realizing as I did so that he was in a sweat.

I held him tight until the shaking subsided, then got out of bed, went around to where I could see his face fully and asked what was going on.

His eyes were very troubled.

He told me he had been assailed by the urge to get up and start a fire. When questioned further, it became clear the urge was to burn the papers he'd been cleaning out of his desk.

Then he added, "It's as if I wanted to burn my whole desk." (He had made the desk for himself.)

I wasn't sure if he was frightened by the possibility of starting a fire or by the thought that he wanted to destroy the desk he had so lovingly created. I was reminded right then of the urge that had gripped him the evening he'd *had* to get his wedding band off.

Ed said that talking about the urge—indeed talking *through* it—helped.

The troubled look was still in his eyes so, to lighten the mood, I suggested we have a shredding-the-papers party.

He gave a wan smile, then, clearly exhausted, got back in bed and was soon asleep.

I couldn't sleep after that. I knew I should probably contact Dr. G about one of the medications I had heard can cause hallucinations.

What had happened that night was clearly in another category from seeing imaginary worms. Yet, it also seemed to me this was very much related to the unraveling. As if not only cleaning out papers and unfinished repairs, or removing one's wedding ring, but also destroying what one had created could help one's soul and spirit find release.

The next morning at breakfast I asked Ed, "What are you afraid of?"

He remembered what had happened the night before, all of it, and my suggestion of a paper-shredding-party. it wasn't as though he'd moved out of an altered state of mind and left it behind.

I asked again, "What are you afraid of?"

"Losing you." He looked sad as he said those words.

I was unable to say anything after giving him a long hug. It didn't feel right to simply repeat things I had heard in the past about never losing those you love who die. I *had* connected with people I, and we, had loved who had died. Ed knew of those connections. And some of them were still ongoing. But this was different. It was as though the losses Ed, and I, had experienced together over the past 12 years, little by little, then faster and faster, were coming down to one big final erasure. *This* body of his, *this* life of his, *this* life we'd lived together in *these* times, they were all coming to an end. I was still here, but he knew he soon would not be here.

Right then I felt, from Ed, the preciousness of physical incarnation in a way I'd never felt it before. Now, writing about it, I have to thank him for that. Being able to be here on our beautiful earth in a body, and with someone you love who is also in a body: that is truly a gift! As I said once to a friend, "It's nice, and it's exciting being able to converse with subtle and spiritual beings, but… it's even more wonderful when you can touch and hug the person you're conversing with."

Ed was grieving—and he knew it.

He told Laurel he was grieving the fact he wouldn't get to see his grandchildren grow up.

He grieved over complicated family situations he felt he hadn't been able to resolve.

He grieved because he didn't feel he had anything more to live for." (That was a painful one to have to listen to.)

He grieved over trips we hadn't been able to take.

He grieved over changes that were occurring in the school he had started.

He found the condition of our country deeply, persistently, painfully grievous.

It feels important that I add here that my own grief didn't just come out in the tears I've mentioned. It came out a few times as anger, and it *always* took me by surprise. Here's a description of one such moment from my journal. Such moments did not happen often, this particular time was one of the worst.

I was so ashamed last night at how angry I was at Ed. He broke the TV remote control again as he fumbled with it so we were unable to get into the science program (Planet Earth) I wanted to watch. The old feeling of wanting something really badly and having, yet again, to put my want aside, try to figure out the way through another mess or mix-up, shove down the disappointment.

He was stunned by my anger –I was too. And I thought I was getting pretty good at swallowing the impatience, irritation, disappointment.

Another glass or plate broken.

Another clogged toilet (so bad we had to get the plumber.)

Another moment of awful noises: the shuffling over the kitchen floor, the chewing, the slurping. And I'm supposed to be deaf, for God's sake!

The slouching...

My anger was directed right then <u>at</u> him. It was unfair, unjustified, uncalled for.

Beneath it all was the anger, this burning rage at the PD being so relentless, so consuming. It felt like a foul constipation in my own body, a clogging up of my love, a hurtfulness that is not, <u>must not worm its way into me and become me</u>. Because I could lose myself if that happened.

In the evening of March 14th Craig, who lives across the street from us and had appeared many times exactly when Ed or I needed a hand, came to dinner. His wife was away for the weekend, and Ed seemed glad it was just the three of us as Craig is a quiet guy who prefers listening to talking.

Ed's legs were extremely rigid. Craig immediately offered an arm to help him get to the table and into his chair.

There was light banter about crazy neighbors, dogs, stealing stones for stone walls, bears passing through, and the coming of spring.

I had just brought out the dessert. I knew Craig loves ice cream and was scooping out a helping for him when Ed suddenly stood up and declared, "I want to go home!"

He began to wobble precariously, so Craig and I jumped up and caught him by the arms.

I wasn't sure just what Ed meant. "Do you want to go up to bed?" I asked.

"I want to go home," Ed repeated, though a bit less emphatically.

Craig and I exchanged a look but didn't say anything.

Then Ed sat down again and asked for his ice cream.

Part Three

Craig went home shortly after dessert that night of March 14 and I helped Ed upstairs and into bed. After I'd cleaned up, done the dishes, and taken Tucker for a short stroll down the road in the dark, I joined Ed in bed. He was already asleep.

Around 11:30 pm I woke in a sweat. I was gulping the air, could barely breathe and was dizzy. No tears or anything, just this weird gulping.

Downstairs in the kitchen I poured myself a tumbler of orange juice (my quick pick-up) and sat down in the darkened living room. I didn't drink the orange juice because of the strange breathing, wasn't sure the juice would stay down.

Though this had never happened to me before, I believe I was having a panic attack.

I wondered if I should try calling 911 or Craig on the TTY but didn't want to be seen in my nightgown. More importantly, I couldn't imagine what would happen to Ed if I was taken to the hospital. I sat there in the dark, hands folded over my heart, shut my eyes and concentrated on slowly trying to slow my breathing.

In and out, in and out, deep and deeper, out and further out.

And my breathing *did* slow.

Then I was suddenly chilly, so wrapped myself in the lap blanket on the sofa.

I next visualized myself in two different places—sanctuaries I'd found—that were important to me when I was younger, both outdoors. First one, then the other. I went into the details of these places as though there: a path, a stream, trees, rocks, moss and so on.

That slowed my breathing further, and I decided I could make it through the night.

Back upstairs I squeezed a couple of drops of the Bach Rescue Remedy under my tongue and went back to bed. Ed was still asleep.

I didn't tell him what had happened when he woke later to go the bathroom, or in the morning when giving him his medications.

I am sharing all of this because, looking back later, I came to the conclusion my body was warning me that Ed and I were coming to a major junction.

It was one of those mornings when Ed drifted off again after taking his medications, so I went on with my day. It felt like a usual everyday day, despite the experience of the night before.

Around 11:30 am Ed came downstairs in his pajamas and settled in the living room. I brought him coffee and a bowl of granola. His movements were usually more fluid in the morning than at any other time during the day, so I was startled when he suddenly put the bowl of granola on the floor, stood up, rigid as a door post, reached for the walker and began to fall over.

I grabbed him, steadied him and asked if he wanted to go to the bathroom.

He nodded but was unable to push the walker forwards.

I tried to help him get going but he was completely frozen, like a block of ice. His rumpled early morning hair looked altogether disheveled, his unshaven cheeks gave him a sunken look, his mouth was half open, his eyes unfocused.

My heart sank: I *knew* I'd reached the point when I could no longer help him physically. My body had warned me the night before. Ed's body was saying, "Enough!"

I asked Ed to sit again, in fact, pushed him down back onto the sofa and ran to the TTY to call Craig. I asked if he could please come over and help me make a decision. Craig said he'd be right over.

When Craig arrived, I told him Ed was too rigid to walk to the bathroom, but we did get him into the back hall.

By then I'd asked Craig to please tell me if he thought I should call 911. He nodded even before I'd finished my sentence and I saw the relief on his face.

Craig got out his cell phone, spoke with the operator, made the connection. He and I made small talk in the back hall before the ambulance came, Ed perched silently on the one chair back there, the walker beside him. I also filled a canvas bag with items I knew Ed would need: his medications and bathroom items, socks, sweatshirt and snacks because I knew how hungry he could get.

A young policeman and a town selectman (who it turned out had been here before when Ed had had a choking episode) arrived first. Then the ambulance with the first responders. It took four men to get Ed onto the stretcher and into the ambulance. My other clear memory of then is of Robin, the young woman who helped me with house cleaning, striding rapidly up our driveway, anxious to see what was going on and if she could help. She and her family had come to take a walk in the nearby sanctuary just when the ambulance pulled into our driveway. I told her Ed was having difficulty moving. What I saw on her face was how much more serious it all looked to her than that. I reassured her we were okay, got into our car and followed the ambulance to the hospital.

For long time I'd been wanting to go on a retreat by myself. I felt the need to step away from the caregiving in order to hear my own thoughts and feelings more clearly. I applied twice to spend three or four days at a monastery. Both reservations had to be canceled, the first because of the bombing on the day of the Boston Marathon, the second a few years later when I had the flu. I know I *could* have taken time away, our girls had offered to come and stay with their father, but I didn't take them up on it. Why not? Two reasons: it didn't feel right going off by myself when Ed couldn't do the same. It's not as though I sat at home all day with him. I swam frequently during the week, took long walks with the dog, was in a care givers support group, did volunteer work and attended a weekly pastel class. Ed had PT, a PD choral group, and we both went to PD dance class every Tuesday, a highlight of our week. When I described the second monastery reservation to Ed, he said how much he would like to do that. But I didn't want us to go together, and it wasn't at all clear (we both agreed on this) how he could do it on his own. (Ed did in 2019 get two nights away with his two brothers at the home of his eldest brother, and that was very important to him and wonderful. As for me: I went to the circus! Not much of a "retreat," for sure!)

The other reason was easy and simple: I love our home. Not just the house itself but the land, trees, gardens, rocks, birds, wild animals, wind, sky, clouds, stars. There's always something to see here. My inner allies are here. When Ed went into the hospital that Sunday in March, the retreat I'd wanted came to me!

We had an awful afternoon in the ER that March 15th waiting to see the first available doctor. We were assigned a brash nurse who said Ed could not take his medications when he always took them because he hadn't yet seen the doctor. Furthermore, he couldn't take the medications I'd brought because they hadn't been prescribed by the ER doctor. (The pill box we'd always used, which I'd grabbed on the way out of our house, was taken away.) In addition, the list I gave the nurse of the medications I'd given Ed that morning differed from the list that I described Ed following the day before. This was because Dr. G had told me, by email, to make a small change in the late afternoon of the day before. He thought this change might address the extreme rigidity. The nurse couldn't make sense of this change and, at one point, snapped at me to shut up and just answer her questions with a "yes" or "no" rather than, "I need to explain that yesterday…" It was **so** frustrating! Ed lay ramrod straight on the bed in the dismal hospital gown, unshaven, his eyes rather unfocused with, hauntingly at moments, the strange darkness in them.

In addition to the issue over the meds, I was aware of the nurse talking about me behind her hand, when two other nurses came in and out. I knew she was telling them I was deaf. It's happened so often, it's pretty obvious when it's happening.

"For God's sake, can you PLEASE get a warm blanket for my husband!" Was the closest I came to snapping back at her.

She *did* get the blanket.

And I *did* thank her.

When the doctor finally came, over an hour later—though it seemed like a whole day later—Ed was dozing off. Actually, interestingly, he didn't seem the worse for not having had the PD medications he was "supposed" to have taken six hours earlier. Goes to show how thoroughly we can give ourselves over to routines. He'd devoured all the snacks I'd brought. I can't remember if I'd brought my iPad along and had let our girls know where we were. Craig may well have called them. I do remember feeling, as I ran a comb through

34

Ed's thinning hair to make him look a bit more civilized, as though we were in a half-way place. Half-way between him leaving our warm home and being submerged in a cold, sterile, colorless, country.

The doctor was young—refreshingly so—and apologetic for taking so long reaching us. It helped to calm *me* to describe to him the events that led to the 911 call and to see he was listening, really listening, and was sympathetic. Ed became a person with a history, not just a body on the bed. Throughout all the hospital visits that followed, I found it scary leaving Ed in the hands of others without any form of identification on him other than the plastic bracelet on his wrist. No wallet, no driver's license with photo, no insurance card, no organ donor card, no cell phone, no wedding band. Suppose Ed got confused and disoriented and his speech wasn't clear? (That had happened briefly now and then in the last six months.) Suppose the people he was with somehow got confused and lost the thread of his particular entry into where he was? (A surgeon had by mistake come very close to operating on my healthy, not my injured, knee some years before.) These feelings and observations made me acutely aware of what I call our outermost identity. This outermost identity being as important and precious as our innermost identity. I see it as a major thread in one's incarnation—both before one passes over and afterwards. The other major thread being our innermost identity, our soul, as Tom speaks of it. The two being absolutely essential to our not unraveling altogether.

The ER doctor checked Ed's eyes, ears, mouth and heart. He admitted he wasn't familiar with PD, but I knew we were being taken seriously. Within twenty or thirty minutes he had admitted Ed to the hospital, rather than releasing him, and had explained Ed would be observed by a neurologist and physical therapists who would determine the next steps to get Ed rehabilitated, then home again. He also explained that Ed would remain in the ER until a room was ready for him, and they would keep an eye on him if I wanted to go home to rest.

Ed urged me to go home. Home I went to our mutt, Tucker, who needed to go out, and to Ed's unfinished breakfast, his pile of clothes from the night before on the chair in the bathroom, his socks and shoes on the floor, the unmade bed and the half empty glass of water on his bedside shelf.

Ed was in the hospital for two days. No more than one visitor was allowed to see Ed at a time. What I remember most clearly are: a very pregnant Black nurse who looked the other way when Christa joined me, knowing that we needed to be together when we visited Ed: the strong, young physical therapist who held Ed up until he could find his balance and stand on his own feet: and the neurologist.

This neurologist was evidently a bit older than Dr. G and more experienced. He quite literally tore the shades off my eyes. After greeting me, he asked if Ed had ever been diagnosed with Lewy Body Dementia, adding he was puzzled not to find any mention of that condition in Ed's file.

Dr. G had never used the term, Lewy Body Dementia, but I knew immediately what this man was talking about. Two friends of ours had died from it: one had PD, the other didn't. The one with PD had gone through a rapid and dangerous decline. I say "dangerous" because he was prone to climbing out the windows of whatever house he was in, usually at night, and wandering off down the road, in the middle of the road. Wherever he was staying, the police had to get him back to safety and he wouldn't always comply.

In that minute all Ed's odd behavior of the previous six months came into focus for me: the repeated messing-up of his own cleaning-up efforts, walking around with one sock and shoe on one foot, taking off his pants in the middle of the day, playing with nail clippers and scissors in a manner that made me uncomfortable (as if he wanted to cut up his fingers), the more combative language, the way he'd snap at me out of the blue, the anxieties ("Someone is after our land…"), the "worms," the urge to start the fire, the strange dark look in his eyes.

Suddenly there was a name for it, a sort-of pattern in it, and very likely an approaching end or—if the people around him weren't alert—a possible crash!

Yet there was a "yet" in it for me: I wasn't about to accept this definite unraveling as an inevitable and final end of his life. I could still see him in his eyes. Christa could too, and we both heard him, and his playful humor in the gentlemanly way he interacted with the nursing and medical staff. His soul was still very much there.

At this point Ed began asking, "What's the plan?" Every day, several times a day, and later in the nursing home also, he would inquire, even beg us to find out, "What's the plan?" Meaning, "Why am I where I am? What's going on? Where am I going?" We both, and Laurel also, when she joined us, repeatedly explained to him that the medical staff was trying to figure out how to help him get beyond the freezing-up so he could be at home. But I knew Ed was asking about *much* more than just that. I heard an echo of my father's persistent question during the weeks before he passed over, "*Where* am I?"

"The plan" according to the kind care team overseeing his possible discharge was, as just mentioned, to loosen up Ed's limbs through concentrated physical therapy and possible shifts in the medications, to get him moving again. All agreed Ed needed rehabilitation in a nursing home setting for about two weeks (about the amount of time Medicare would cover). And when he was discharged from the nursing home I'd have to have 24/7 care in place, because I couldn't do it all on my own. The girls and I were relieved by their acknowledgement of the fact that I would need help, but I was puzzled because the focus was entirely on Ed's acute physical challenges with really no mention of his psychological condition.

When I emailed Dr. G asking why he hadn't said anything to us about Lewy Body Dementia, he said (in effect): "We all know he's in late stage PD with dementia. At this point it doesn't really matter whether it's called dementia or Lewy Body Dementia, because those conditions affect the same part of the brain." I accepted this explanation. It didn't seem worth being upset with him in any way. Besides I hadn't really described Ed's odd behavior to him in detail nor spoken with him about the hallucinations. And hadn't Ed seemed pretty spry at the end of his last appointment? However, I do now believe it can be helpful to those on the PD journey who are trying to follow the twists and turns of their own personal itinerary, to know about the differences between PD dementia and Lewy Body Dementia. I am certain Ed had Lewy Body Dementia, that it hastened his decline and made it quite a bit more extreme and dramatic than it would have been if he had just had dementia. I think he knew, when he was wrestling with the term "cognitive decline" that there was more in store for him than just that. Ed and I met enough people with

PD during the last 12 years for me to say this: I also believe—with all my heart—that dementia or Lewy Body Dementia is *not* automatically in the cards for every person who gets a PD diagnosis.

The hospital care team gave me the names of three nursing homes in town for us to check out and list by preference. I already knew of them and which was my first choice. It was the one where a close friend of ours had passed over, but there was no room for Ed. This turned out to be a blessing, and, for me, a reminder that I was no longer in charge of all the details of Ed's life. Not that I necessarily had been before, just that I was no longer the main contact person in connection to his physical well-being. In fact, Ed's caregiving "team" on this side had more than doubled overnight! I'm not just speaking here of medical, nursing and home help and caregiving assistance, but of our daughters stepping forward immediately. We three quickly became a team. From this point on one or the other, sometimes both together, was/were with me at all the main junctions in the last month of Ed's life. By "junctions" I mean moments when major decisions had to be made or when Ed was being moved physically from one place to another. I felt, and still feel, incredibly lucky in this regard and wish the same for anyone who finds herself in the situation I found myself in.

Laurel, who drove up from and back to DC four times within two months (an 8-hour drive each way), oversaw research into nursing homes. She did this because it quickly became clear *we* were expected to do it ourselves, especially if we hoped to keep Ed close to home. COVID was, like a fire, flaring up right then in western Massachusetts, and there was a rush to find "beds" for people in all kinds of situations.

Christa, who lives three hours away, was the main contact person on the phone with the doctors, nurses, physical therapists and case workers. Not that Laurel and I didn't talk with some of them too, just that it made sense that it would be easier for them this way. (I myself can't talk on the phone but did, later, FaceTime with the last doctor Ed had when being hospitalized.)

And I did what I could to keep track of the medications Ed had been on and was being advised by Dr. G and others to take, because I was so shaken by the nurse in the ER when Ed first went into the hospital. All the nurses after her were excellent and easy to communicate with, but that jarring experience reminded me of tragic medical mix-ups I'd heard about in the past. In addition, Dr. G was still suggesting Ed try the medication for cognitive decline that he had spoken of at our last appointment. The medication described in the flyer Dr. G handed me with the healthy-looking couple holding hands. The very first description in the list of possible side effects from that medication was: there is a higher chance of death in older adults who take this drug for mental problems caused by dementia.

Looked at one way, I knew Ed was on his way out, and he knew it too, so....? Yet every fiber of my being was saying, "NO! This medication is *not* for Ed!"

When Ed went into the nursing home, I remained clear on this NO although Dr. G continued to speak of it. My understanding of this now is that this medication *could* have interfered in some way with the passage of his soul out of his body.

Put another way, I was being told the most important thing I could do was to stay attentive not only to whatever Ed's soul was trying to communicate but to the intuitions in my own soul from and about him. I could no longer talk with him in person, with words or touch, the way we had throughout our married life, but we were still very much connected. As outer physical help with Ed's unraveling body came forwards, it was important I step back, away from him physically into the silence, the retreat, being made available to me at home, in order to pay close and closer attention to Ed's inner journey.

On St. Patrick's Day, Christa and I heard of the first reported COVID case at a nursing home in town. It was at the one that had been my first choice, the one we'd been told was full.

Christa and I had agreed that morning that we would go together to the hospital and take turns visiting with Ed, as they were strictly enforcing the "one visitor only" rule. I went first and, while greeting Ed, was informed by a smiling case manager that a bed had been found at another nursing home, and Ed would be discharged within the hour. Ed's eyes lit up, "the plan" was on!

I emailed Christa, then Laurel, the news, assembled Ed's belongings so he'd be ready to go when the ambulance transport team arrived, and went back to the main lobby of the hospital hoping to see Christa before she went in for her time with her father. No sign of her, so I went outside for some air and exercise.

I was circling back to the hospital main entrance when Christa emailed me to go to the back door of the ER immediately, as Ed was on his way to the ambulance. Rather than go around the outside of the building I went straight through, came out the back door, and there was Christa running towards me tears streaming down her face.

"We won't be able to see him..." she sobbed.

She had just gotten a call from the nursing home warning us they had gone into lockdown down an hour earlier because of COVID. Ed was welcome there, we weren't.

This was the first I'd heard of lockdowns, and it made no sense at all to me. Ed was already confused; how was he going to retain *any* mental stability if he was among complete strangers? As I felt it, Ed badly needed people he knew, needed his family, if he was to be safe, comfortable, truly cared for.

Minutes later Ed appeared on the stretcher, two first responders, both masked, accompanying him. Christa and I ran over to explain the situation to him as they began lifting him into the back of the ambulance. He looked totally baffled.

"You're going to the nursing home," Christa and I both told him. "We won't be able to visit you because there's a lock-down, no visitors are allowed at all, not even family."

He and I stared at each other.

Ed could see I'd been crying and asked me very directly, "Do you want me to resist?"

I almost laughed because it was such an improbable thing for him to be able to do—he was so thin and weak-- and because it was such a brave thing to offer. I'll never forget the way he said that.

But I shook my head, because the three men in uniform, standing there listening, were waiting for us to say good-bye so they could get him where he was going. Christa told them we would go directly to the nursing home as I needed to sign some papers.

To shorten the story: Christa and I learned when we reached the nursing home that Ed's room was on the ground floor and his bed was by the window. We immediately went to see if that was the case, and there he was sitting in a wheelchair at the foot of the bed the nurse was about to help him into. His face brightened when we saw us. We both waved, blew kisses and gestured we would be back soon.

Every day, at least twice a day, between March 17th and April 3rd, even if it was raining or snowing, I made window visits to Ed at the nursing home. Christa accompanied me once or twice before heading home. Tucker, our mutt, almost always came when I discovered the nursing home lounge, a few rooms down from Ed's bedroom, with its longer, larger windows. There was a patio outside the lounge with metal garden chairs so I'd sit in one of the chairs, a blanket drawn tight around me, or an umbrella overhead, Tucker beside me, inches from Ed in his wheelchair, parked on the other side of the glass door out to the patio.

At first Ed tried to open the door, to get out, to be with us. The nurses had to restrain him while trying to explain the lockdown situation. I could see it made no sense to him and often departed earlier than planned so as not to aggravate him further.

I knew that the main problem in visiting with him this way was that he couldn't hear me. Seeing each other was great, not being able to talk with words or by way of touch –we'd put our hands up, his hands over mine on the window pane as if we could touch –was exceedingly painful. I'd always been the deaf one, now he was deaf.

I brought along legal pads and magic markers, wrote in big letters, and held what I'd written up against the window. Sometimes the light from outside made him squint or shift about in the wheelchair but, fortunately, he could still read and comprehend what he was reading.

I'd lip read his responses and scribble back my reply, often feeling as though I couldn't write fast enough—meaning fast enough to hold his attention. I found the thought of the number of words we'd always used to communicate on a daily basis astonishing. It was like opening a refrigerator and realizing we'd normally eaten quite a bit, and now, now more than half of the food inside was old, dried out, stale.

To maintain the connection, to keep the conversation going, I asked questions which could be answered with a Yes or No.

Did you have a good night? "No." (Most of the time.)

Do you like your roommate? "No—he watches TV all day, the TV is on full blast."

Are you aware of the news? He wasn't sure how to answer that one. Not knowing how to begin describing what was going on in the world, I didn't say any more but decided I'd get him a copy of *The New York Times* later that day. And some of his favorite Reese's Peanut Butter cups. Anything to help him reconnect with life outside that window. I thought that, even though I knew everything was still unraveling.

When I asked Ed about the physical therapist and nurses, he became more animated. Did he like them? "Yes!" I saw from his face that they cared. He wanted me to meet one of the nurses, a gentle, older lady with shy smile. I was able to talk with the Physical Therapist through a slightly opened window, and out of that came the idea that Ed might be able to converse with me and other outdoor visitors and family at a distance, via FaceTime. Laurel and Christa had also suggested this. So, when bringing Ed's clothing and toiletries to the nursing home, I included the iPad the family had given him for Christmas.

Ed had been totally frustrated throughout the fall by his PC and, with the help of a young tech-savy neighbor, had tried to learn to manage simple email exchanges and daily access to PD websites and news sources. But, between fumbling fingers and short-term memory gaps, things had gotten worse and worse. Ed was ready, although at first a bit skeptical when he got the iPad, and realized he'd have to learn a whole new set of steps to get and stay online. The girls and the son-in-law who had researched the options and set things up for Ed were incredibly patient when giving directions. And Ed *had* tried FaceTime, and, like me, was astonished by it, before he was hospitalized.

However, the sad, and difficult part of turning to FaceTime was that he was soon trying to call the three of us, and some others also, any time of day or night. He was pressing the buttons to get *someone*, indeed any one of us, without really knowing exactly how to follow the steps not only of connecting online but connecting one-on-one. I was shocked by his desperation to connect. Laurel or Christa, often emailed me to say, "Daddy wants to talk… I'm in the middle of a business meeting" or "I tried calling him back, but he didn't respond." To me the constant calling, or trying to call, sounded like a variation of the question he'd been asking before he went into the hospital, "What's the plan?" Telling the nurses exactly when we each could connect with him on FaceTime helped somewhat—helped make the connections more orderly—but then he wasn't always in the mood to talk during those times.

Then, as though tuning into the political energies surging around in the ether, he began to talk in the tone of conspiracy theories: some dangerous commune was after Christa, some crazy person was after our land, when I came back that evening, when no one was looking, he would escape from "them" with me. I could see he wanted to get out but also, in the darkness of his look, saw the advance of the Lewy Body Dementia. All of this is not to say we didn't respond to what he said. We were continually telling him the doctor and therapists expected him to reach a certain level of mobility, then he would be able to leave. We told him, too, that I was getting our house ready for this time: a hospital bed, a wheelchair, a ramp for the wheelchair, hand grips in the bathroom and hallway, a special shower, a commode, a wonderful helper named Lisa who had voluntarily gone through quarantine so she could be with us when he came home.

Two completely different images stand out in my memory from this time when Ed was in the nursing home.

In the first, I realized he was tied to the wheelchair.

It happened like this:

I arrived at the lounge window one afternoon with Tucker but didn't find Ed in his usual spot near the window either fiddling with his iPad, staring at a newspaper or magazine, or looking out in my direction. A glance into his room told me he wasn't there.

I returned to the lounge window and tapped on it. By then most of the nurses knew who I was and why I was there. One of them came over, and said Ed was now being "parked" near the nurse's station at the back of the room (when she said that I recognized the back of his head.) She then wheeled him over by the window to visit with me.

There was an anxious look on his face. Ed tried to stand when he saw me but couldn't because of something attached to the back of his sweatshirt.

The nurse pushed him down and explained, as of the day before he'd been wanting to stand but was very wobbly. In fact, the previous night he shot up and the nurses *just* caught him before he toppled over, in the same way Craig and I had caught him when he had suddenly stood and declared, *"I want to go home!"*

"A nurse can't be with him *every* minute," she said apologetically, and returned to her station.

"I *hate* this," Ed said trying to yank his sweatshirt free of whatever it was fastened to.

"They're afraid you'll fall and hurt yourself."

He scowled.

It was not a good, nor a long visit

The other memory is of another dark moment when I was visiting at the lounge window and, to lighten the mood, began singing the old folksong:

You are my sunshine, my only sunshine
You make me happy when skies are grey
You'll never know, dear, how much I love you
Please don't take my sunshine away...

Ed was immediately right with me, joining in. When I couldn't recall the third or fourth stanza, he switched over easily with me onto "a bicycle built for two," then from there into *Peace I Ask of Thee of O River*. When I put my hands up against the windowpanes on the lower part of the door before leaving, Ed, on his side, put his over mine. When I put the imprint of a kiss on the windowpane near his nose, he imprinted his kiss on the other side, on top of mine.

It was abundantly clear that music was, then, the best way to reach Ed, to call him out of the darker moments. Friends sang with him. And one freezing cold afternoon, the leader of the PD choral group he was in, a lovely young woman, a soprano, who happened to be very pregnant, joined me on the patio with one of her colleagues to sing for and with him. The two ladies sang, laughed, gently teased Ed, and asked at the end of their visit if there was a last song he wanted to hear.

I had to turn away to hide my tears as they sang *Amazing Grace*.

Part Four

When Ed was in the nursing home I saw him twice a day 20 or 25 minutes a day. And sometimes, as when there were visitors who weren't sure how to find him at the window, more than twice a day. Though it was late March, it was often wet and cold on the patio, even if I wore hat, mittens, boots, parka and a blanket around my shoulders.

Ed was much annoyed at first at not being able to open the door to get outside to join Tucker and me. He fumbled with the doorknob and, through gestures when the nurses weren't looking, we pantomimed his escape. Heck, he would tear the knob right out of the socket! There would even be a hole *this big* when he got it out! (Thumbs and forefingers together he showed me the size of the hole.) I grinned and offered both hands and arms as imaginary support for when he came out.

During these moments, FaceTime on iPads, and words scribbled on paper and held up on the windowpane, were left behind. What we needed to say to one another was better expressed through the immediacy of gestures, movements, facial expressions, "looks." And there was a fair amount of "us" versus "them" (meaning the medical authorities). That was actually, at moments, fun.

However, startled by the force of what Ed was trying to express and mindful of the dark side of Lewy Body Dementia, which I had seen the night he woke wanting to start a fire, I didn't encourage "talk" of this sort. I mimed back, not very successfully, myself driving him home when they released him.

"**WHEN**?" demanded his eyes.

As he was unable to read the words on my lips, I wrote out, "Soon...... I hope."

But, as with young children, "soon" can become a torment, not a promise.

It hurt greatly having to watch Ed become resigned to being on the other aside of the window. It solidified the feeling of separation, of him becoming part of life elsewhere, life I couldn't share with him. Where did they put his clothing? What did the bathroom he used look like? Did they ever take him into other rooms than the ones I could see through the windows? I had no idea.

It was and it wasn't strange being alone in our house, on retreat, while Ed was in the nursing home. It was strange because I was still geared to medication and meal schedules, to making sure Ed got to appointments and to waking when he woke in the middle of the night. And suddenly none of that was necessary. Not having to think about cooking at, say, exactly 5:30 pm was marvelous. Scrambled eggs, or a baked potato with cheese on top, or, as I discovered later—down the road—two coconut popsicles, was plenty for me.

On the other hand, this retreat *wasn't* strange because Ed was very much with me, and I don't mean simply in thought. I was not surprised when I got to the nursing home window in the morning and learned from the nurses he'd been agitated part of the night. Up the hill, five miles away, I'd felt the agitation at 2:00 am. Nor was I surprised when nurses and doctors told me now and then Ed had suddenly, out of the blue, asked for "Claire..." I could hear him. My inner response, at a distance, to what I sensed coming from him was usually brief and varied according to where I was at that moment, from "I'm at the post office..." to "Love you..."

This is *not* to say I was constantly aware of Ed. Other things, like getting the house ready for his return, connecting with the doctors, updating family and friends, and of course the news, were much on my mind. I also felt vistas opening within myself that I hadn't been responsive to before. Put simply, it was as though, my focus up until then had been so entirely on Ed's physical well-being that I'd stopped seeing how tall the trees round our home had grown, how commanding the shapes of the rocks in the garden are, and how there were mole hills *everywhere*. In the past, in the late winter and early spring, the burrowing moles had greatly annoyed Ed and me—they sure messed up our yard. But now I had to smile. Those moles were *so* busy! Every day, when I went to and returned from the nursing home, I saw new mounds had popped up, reminiscent of the maze puzzle books our younger grandkids had loved to race through with crayons.

John Gardner, who played an important part in my introduction to the work of Rudolf Steiner and had been my mentor and close friend for over 30 years, and was also a friend of Ed, had once told me the etheric bodies of married couples can become finely interwoven and when one partner is very ill and/or dies the surviving spouse can experience etheric disturbance, even physical pain. (This can also happen, John had added, to close friends and to parents and their children.)

The etheric body, according to Steiner, also known as the life body, is, "that which animates a living being, bringing movement and metamorphosis to what would otherwise be inherent matter. It is a body of forces rather than substance." I'd felt the truth of John's observation many times during the years Ed struggled with Parkinson's. I was able to pick up on some of Ed's thoughts and his emotional and physical discomforts, even if we weren't together in person. I described this to some extent in my book *Rolling With The Waves: Our Parkinson's Journey* (published by Lorian Press in 2019.)

Now this phenomenon was, for me, becoming even more pronounced, and it wasn't just limited to Ed being unable to sleep, or being agitated, or physically constrained by his body or being tied to the wheelchair. There were moments when I sensed Ed was struggling with very definite emotions, and these, I also sensed, were important because they presented a way for me to remain in touch with him, even to travel *with* him as he made his way towards death.

The best example I can give had to do with powerful feelings of regret. They were there in the morning when I woke. These feelings were similar to the grief described earlier but were several degrees more specific. Rather than a general feeling of sadness or disappointment there was some shame, contrition, and self-reproach. At first, I took them to be *my* regrets. I *did* have some feelings of regret, bordering on guilt, that I hadn't done everything possible to prevent Ed from having to go to the hospital, then the nursing home, but, overall, I knew I'd done the best I could at the moment. And I was regretful when remembering times when I'd been impatient because of the PD or had lost my temper.

However, when I visited Ed at the window, it became clear from his facial expressions, despondent hand movements, and verbal comments, he *was* feeling regretful about various situations in his past. I'm not going to go into those situations because they were his private business. Will just say that I felt the overall mood or thrust of these regrets—if Ed had been able to articulate what was weighing on him—might have come out in the form of a question: "Did I live my life as thoughtfully, creatively and lovingly as I could have?"

Ed's distress right then made life—not his life specifically but life here on earth—suddenly seem very short. How *can* one possibly squeeze everything one wants, hopes or longs to do into a life? Is it actually "normal" (that weird word) to feel one has fallen short? And might regret —with that feeling of falling short—actually be the kernel of a seed being planted in the depths of the soul, the seed of wanting another chance, another life?

As these thoughts passed through me while I drove down the hill every day to the nursing home, then back up the hill to my hermitage, I felt how the movement of the life that Ed and I had shared was, paradoxically, changing right then from unraveling to reweaving. And actually—considering the circumstances—a lot more than mere unraveling was occurring. Ed was literally being ripped out of not just his home but his family and community because of our very limited and proscribed access to him. The reweaving for him, as I see it now, meant having to accept the care and good intentions of strangers and strange places, having to let go of familiar forms of communicating, having to yield to life as it pushed him closer and closer to death. And the reweaving, for me, meant being with him as fully as I could outwardly and even more so inwardly. My prayer for him then was that he be filled with courage; "Courage from the hand of God" as expressed in a verse I sent his way. I envisioned a cocoon of blue light around him. And prayed that those on the other side who were awaiting him "protect, border and salute" him because, golly, he looked so very alone sitting in the wheelchair by the window.

In terms of the physical rehabilitation Ed had been sent to get at the nursing home, Ed did look better. A bit less rigid but, at the same time, clearly now very dependent on the wheelchair. He still had to be tied to it because of the recurring need to stand up. And when he stood up, always suddenly, forcefully, as if being called, he couldn't keep his balance and would crash over if not caught.

This abrupt standing looked, to me, like a mysteriously metaphorical act. (I learned later the PD experts call this "postural instability" and it's often a predominant feature of late stage PD.) It was as if Ed was not merely trying to be upright but was trying to righten himself right out of his physically battered body into a place of new strength and balance. Though it was a headache for others having to keep an eye on him—and I knew this job would likely land on me when he was released from the nursing home—I also, inwardly, felt the urge to applaud him.

A day or two before Ed was released, the nursing home informed us the first case of COVID had been detected in their midst, the infected patient had been immediately isolated, and all who were staying there, lived there, or worked there were being isolated and tested. They wouldn't tell us if Ed had been anywhere near this person but said, until we knew the result of his test, he would have to be isolated at home for at least two weeks. In addition, those who took care of him should wear masks and gloves, wash their hands frequently and limit their contact with others. That meant myself, Laurel who had joined me to help bring Ed home, and Lisa, the wonderful caregiver who landed, as though through providence, on our doorstep at the exact right moment. (I later learned the person with COVID who set this wave of anxious vigilance in motion around us—and this was my first exposure to it—was the wife of a dear friend in my caregiver's support group. Trish was in her 90s and had Alzheimer's. She was in a different wing of the nursing home from Ed; he was never anywhere near her, and she recovered from the virus.)

The COVID twist made things quite a bit more difficult. Though I myself was more rested than I'd been when Ed went into the nursing home, and was certain Lisa was going to be a big help, I was scared. In fact, I was terrified. Even if we had a wheelchair and ramp, one of the guest rooms had been turned into a special room for Ed with a hospital bed, and there was room in the adjoining guest room for

Lisa, care at this level felt like a whole new ball game. And Ed seemed more confused than ever. Would that change when he was back in familiar territory, or had he lost ground to the Lewy Body Dementia when at the nursing home?

Both Laurel and Christa knew me well enough to pick up on my anxiety and insisted I ask Lisa for as much help as possible, especially at night, so I could rest. Then they urged me to look for yet more help, and we agreed the visiting therapists—if these professionals were permitted to come in person to the house—would be an important part of that. It was a "Let's see what happens and go from there..." situation.

Laurel accompanied me in the car to the nursing home, and Ed was wheeled into the lobby. It was the first time we had been together in person in 18 days, since the moment he'd asked if he should resist being taken in the ambulance to the nursing home. His face brightened when he saw Laurel and me. We exchanged hoorays that he was on his way home at last. There was no question he was weaker, thinner, less fully present. Clearly still very much a patient, not a recovered or recovering person. I touched his shoulder but didn't kiss him or take his hand, because of the COVID protocols.

I listened to instructions, signed papers, took the bag of medications and accompanied him on the ride home in the ambulance. Laurel drove the car with the wheelchair and other bags with his clothing and belongings. Ed perked up when he realized the young man in the back of the ambulance with us had a close friend who had graduated from Ed's charter school.

It took both ambulance guys to get Ed into the wheelchair, then up the ramp and into the house. The three of us spent the rest of the day in the living room and out on the patio, with Ed napping either in the wheelchair or the hospital bed.In the early evening, before Lisa arrived, we had supper in his office while watching the news. Then Lisa introduced herself to him and helped him bathe, get into his nightclothes and into bed. Curiously, I don't remember this day very well apart from feeling: first he was glad to be home; and second, the COVID protocols we'd been told to observe were a damn nuisance, an invisible barrier between us. To this day I regret I didn't climb into bed with Ed to give him a good hug and kiss before saying good night. His eyes were asking for that.

The next morning when I went downstairs around 5:00 to see how things were going, Lisa, who'd hardly gotten any sleep and was eager to go home, said Ed had been restless most of the night. I helped him relieve himself, changed his clothing, got him back into bed and he drifted off. When Laurel, who was sleeping in the room over the garage, joined us a few hours later Ed was awake and hungry. I remember the enormous breakfast he ate: a large bowl of oatmeal, several pieces of toast, fruit, scrambled eggs. For a minute I wondered what they'd been feeding him — if anything — in the nursing home.

That Saturday looked as though it was going to be as mild and slow-paced as the day before, with us wheeling Ed between the rooms on the ground floor and briefly outside. He listened to music, leafed through some of the family albums, and Laurel, for a while, set him up with the film, *Pride and Prejudice,* on her computer. I believe it was around this time we got the call saying Ed had tested negative for COVID. That meant I could hug and kiss him. He felt dry, bony and still extremely rigid.

Towards the end of lunch we three began singing, and Ed promptly launched into his favorite song from our Parkinson's dance class:

Some bright morning when this life is over
I'll fly away
To that home on God's celestial shore
I'll fly away

I'll fly away, oh glory
I'll fly away in the morning
When I die hallelujah by and by
I'll fly away

When the shadows of this life have gone
I'll fly away
Like a bird from these prison walls
I'll fly away

I'll fly away, oh glory
I'll fly away in the morning
When I die hallelujah by and by
I'll fly away

Oh how glad and happy when we meet
I'll fly away
No more cold iron shackles on my feet
I'll fly away...

It was the line, "No more cold iron shackles on my feet," that did me in. I cried and cried. *You Are My Sunshine* had Laurel in tears.

The two of us cried, laughed and dabbed at our eyes and noses. Ed watched. He seemed both present, aware of our emotional response to the words, and curiously detached. It was a strange bittersweet moment, a forewarning.

We were having an early supper at the dining room table, Ed in the wheelchair, Laurel and I on either side of him, when he picked up his bowl of ice cream and made as if to eat directly from the bowl with his tongue. Afraid the ice cream would slip out of the bowl and down his face and clothing, I jumped up and the next thing I knew he was standing, pulling away from me—clearly angry at my interference–and had hurled the bowl over his left shoulder. Then he crashed over backwards, away from the wheelchair near the stairs. He just missed hitting his head on the edge of a table near the front door.

Laurel and I leapt to his assistance.

He lay there crumpled while we gently examined one part of his body after another, did his head hurt? His neck? His shoulder? His elbow? His arm? His knee? He shook his head each time and gradually relaxed as he moved out of the uncomfortable heap he'd landed in. We were greatly relieved there didn't appear to be any breaks.

Ed lay on the floor for a while, resting, eyes shut, looking very helpless. We then positioned ourselves on either side to lift him into the wheelchair, but that didn't work. He felt like dead weight. He was way too heavy for us. We were able to get him into what looked like a more comfortable position, sitting upright a bit against the wall, pillows on either side, a blanket around him. I was reluctant to call 911 so soon again.

We decided to wait till Lisa came, certain she would know what to do. Laurel had, by then, called her to ask her to come earlier.

When Lisa arrived, the three of us got Ed back into the wheelchair. Lisa and I cleaned him up, got him into his PJ's, combed his hair, and the four of us settled in the living room. Ed was quiet, obviously fatigued, somewhat docile. I still felt stunned by the anger with which he'd responded when I'd reached for the bowl of ice cream—had I been too bossy or something? I knew Laurel had been stunned too. What had triggered that outburst? What else might happen? At the same time, we knew it was absolutely essential we convey a mood of calm and care.

Lisa had noticed when we were getting Ed into his PJ's how long his toenails were, so she kindly and thoughtfully sat on a stool beside him in the living room and gave him a pedicure while we asked her questions about her family and work. I know he appreciated the pedicure and foot rub she gave him and listened to her life story. Then we got him into bed and after Lisa had told him she'd be on call in the next room, and she and Laurel had said good night, I got a few minutes alone with him.

It felt very strange standing beside the bed—Lisa had put the guard rail up so I couldn't sit down beside Ed—holding his left hand with my two hands, looking into his eyes. I babbled about how great it was having him home, how I'd be wheeling him around on Patten Road so he could say hello to his tree friends, how we'd be getting into a rhythm with physical therapists coming to help him, Lisa would sleep over every couple of nights so I could get my sleep. On some level we both knew none of this was going to happen, but it was important right then to pretend. Why pretend? Because we needed to keep our balance in what we knew, what was familiar, as the unknown pressed down on us.

I kissed Ed, wished him sweet dreams, and turned the light out.

Only three hours later, around 12:30 am, Lisa shook me hard.

Instantly awake, I turned the light on and saw the urgency and fear on her face.

"Get Laurel! GET LAUREL, RIGHT NOW!"

Ed had climbed out of the hospital bed, had made his way to the back hall –God knows how--and was raging mad.

I pulled on my robe, grabbed the processor for my cochlear implant and put it on.

Laurel was sleeping in the room over the garage and I had to go through the back hall to get out the door to get to her.

There was Ed with Lisa holding him as best as she could against the wall. He glared at me. The dark look in his eyes was, as I indicated earlier, **NOT** him. What it was, where it came from, what caused it, I do not know. And still don't know.

I slipped past them and ran to the door leading to Laurel's room. She'd locked it and the lights were out. I banged on the door and yelled for Laurel, but she didn't hear me.

I ran back in, Lisa was still holding Ed against the wall, talking to him, telling him to stop behaving as he was behaving. She warned me he had said he wanted to get a weapon.

I tried reaching Laurel on her phone by way of the TTY (text telephone for the deaf) but she didn't respond. Then I ran out the front door, around to the garage and banged and called for her again.

Back inside the back hall, I looked directly at Ed, as he wrestled with Lisa trying to get out of her grip, and said as forcefully as I could, "**Stop this! You're hurting her, STOP this immediately!**" I meant it through and through. (Ed had often during his life expressed horror and puzzlement, at the violence done to women through rape, other forms of sexual abuse, and on account of domestic dispute and addictions.)

Ed paused and I knew he had heard me. I knew the Ed I knew was back, at least briefly. Later, when in conversation with Christa on the phone, it was evident Ed remembered what had happened, as he expressed remorse. He never said anything to me about this but, in the moment when I knew he had heard me I was aware that, for the first time in my life I had, briefly, been afraid of my husband.

At this point Laurel, who had not only locked the door but

turned her phone off and was sleeping deeply, heard the commotion and came in the back door. She saw right away that her father was behaving strangely. She says he told her he had a knife in the bedroom. Later she checked around the room and found nothing. Ed may have been trying to get to the kitchen when Lisa stopped him. It sounded as though the force that had woken him when he felt compelled to start a fire, was after him again.

With Laurel present, Ed seemed to shrink back into himself. He actually looked smaller. We got him a chair and he sat down, right there, in the back hall. We put a blanket around his shoulders and socks on his feet. It felt important that calm prevail so I got a box of graham crackers, which he always liked to munch on in the evening, and ginger ale for all of us in small glasses.

The family pictures hung on the wall right behind him. It was early morning of the day before our 52nd[h] anniversary, and Ed began talking about our marriage. He gave me the "Tell them your version of how we met" look, as he'd always enjoyed telling and hearing that story, but, right then, I wasn't up to it.

Laurel, Lisa and I exchanged looks: what were we to do? We knew, after all that had happened that evening, we couldn't just put Ed back to bed, and go back to bed ourselves. We knew whatever it was that gripped him was a danger to us and to him.

So we called 911.

Part Five: Reweaving

When he was being taken out the door to the ambulance, Laurel heard her father say, "It's been wonderful—see you later!"

She told me it was said lightly, the way he could say silly, even irrelevant things, every now and then. Ed and I often did that. He was *never* being sarcastic or cynical when he talked this way.

Laurel, Lisa and I followed the ambulance to the hospital. That was the last time I saw Ed in person. Laurel, however, made a point of going in with him to talk with the ER doctor. As Ed was more himself when he left the house, both Lisa and Laurel wanted to be sure the doctor understood Ed had not been himself an hour and a half earlier, had been behaving strangely, violently. Later Laurel described her relief when she realized the young ER doctor heard her, understood what she was saying, and assured her Ed would not be merely examined and sent home.

In the late morning the hospital psychiatrist called to ask if Ed had ever mentioned suicide to me. He hadn't. This doctor then said it was common for people who are suicidal not to tell their spouse. Ed had told him he'd thought about jumping from a bridge in the area where several have taken their lives over the years. While startled by this—didn't Ed and I talk together about pretty much *everything*—I almost laughed aloud. Because, how in the world would Ed—who couldn't walk or drive (I'd taken his car keys away)—have gotten to that bridge? Admittedly, Ed *had* made his way out of the bedroom and into the back hall the night before, after being bound to a wheelchair for half a month, but the thought of him getting himself to that bridge was ludicrous. The doctor added they were looking for an opening in a psychiatric unit where Ed could be evaluated and treated, and within the day had found a spot for him at a medical center two and a half hours eastwards. We were asked to bring a bag of Ed's clothing and some personal belongings to the ER as soon as possible and were reminded we would not be able to visit with him there or

59

where he was being taken. Ed was entirely out of our hands, on his own from then on.

The next day, our anniversary, Ed was transported to the psychiatric unit and the day after, which was his 76th birthday, the nurses sang Happy Birthday to him as we had asked. Laurel and I had made sure the few birthday cards and gifts we had for him were in the bag with his clothing. Later the nurses made a point of showing him in a new fleece pull-over I'd given him when we tried to reach him on FaceTime. He responded to our voices but looked shell-shocked.

A strange week followed. Christa had joined us in the afternoon of the day Ed went back into the hospital. Laurel had to return to her family in DC but, before she left, we three sat down and mapped out everything each of us was going to do, from Laurel exploring nursing home options because Ed, if he was released, wouldn't be able to return to the nursing home he'd been in, to Christa phoning the doctor and nurses daily and letting us know what they had to say, to my being in touch with Dr. G. The week was strange not only because the online photo of the building Ed was in was altogether nondescript but because we had no sense of what was going on. What were they doing with him? Was he in the same room all day? Was he in bed all day? Did he have a window with a view? A roommate? How old were the other patients? We knew little except that the staff was extremely busy.

Christa reassured me the nurses sounded kind and caring. She got their first names so she could ask for and speak with them one-on-one about her father, and they helped arrange FaceTime calls with Ed. One of Ed's brothers and one old friend also tried to make contact with him this way. However, I found those FaceTime calls intolerable. The nurse would prop Ed up with the iPad then leave the room and Ed didn't know how to sit so the camera was on his face. All too often I was simply looking at his forehead, or his hair, unable to see his eyes or read his lips. I couldn't tell if he actually heard me.

Right then and there I sensed that, in order to connect with the Ed I know and love, concentrating on his ailing body, as seen on FaceTime or on disturbing memories of the last couple of months, wasn't the way to go. I needed to find *him*, the healthy core of him.

I'd had practice before in being present with those who are dying or have died, and every experience was different just as every person is different. But, in all of them, it was evident, again and again, whether we're alive or dead, our consciousness can move around quite freely outside of our physical body.

For example, when my father was dying, there was an afternoon when Ed and I were alone with him and he lay silently in bed, eyes shut, then open, then shut again, neither here nor there. As my father didn't appear to be in a state of discomfort, Ed took a break and went out for a walk. I'd been sitting beside my father, reading, and felt the urge to go upstairs to look for a favorite photo of him with my mother. While upstairs I had the feeling he also was upstairs, moving around, though his body was on the bed downstairs in the guest room. I found the photo and sat briefly with it in my hands on the bed in the room that been theirs. I got the inner impression they—my mother and father—were talking about me, even though my mother had passed over 12 years earlier.

A couple of minutes later I went back downstairs to the guest room. My father was awake and talking.

"I think…" he was groping for words, "…. we did the right thing with Claire."

He obviously didn't know, because of the dementia, who I was.

"What do you mean?" I asked.

"Claire lost all her hearing," he replied.

"What happened?" I asked.

"She was very sick…" He sounded worried. "…did …did we do the right thing?"

I took it he was having second thoughts 64 years later about his response to my deafness. It was quite a thought that he was still concerned about something that, to me, had happened long ago. What he was mulling over I don't know, but it seemed important to reassure him.

"I'm certain you did the right thing," I told him, and he drifted off again.

It *was* odd talking about myself in the third person, but, by then I was accustomed not only to him getting people, and past and present, mixed up—in our usual way of seeing things, that is. I was certain his consciousness was moving around outside of his body. And he'd not only been upstairs too when I went up but was in touch with my mother and likely others as well. In addition to moving around the house, he was moving around the different rooms and chapters of his life and may, like Ed, have been working through uncertainties and regrets. Maybe what we call dementia is actually an outer reflection of some inner phase we need to go through in order to transition back into spirit realms. And maybe—it occurs to me right now as I remember the medication Dr. G wanted us to consider using to treat Ed's cognitive decline—maybe some of these medications for people with dementia can mess up a necessary soul process.

What served me best in the effort to find Ed, was the belief that, though he was physically in a strange place among strangers two plus hours away, he might join me as he had for years in our morning time. So, after Christa returned to her home and I was alone again, I sat down each morning "with" Ed. It began with the memory-thought of him in his better days, sometimes arriving before me at our spot, sometimes a few minutes late, usually with his cup of coffee and his reading glasses. I thought of him in his light copper-colored down jacket which he favored inside as well as out, his jeans, his socks and slippers. He had his chair, I had mine. Tucker always joined us, occasionally at our feet, but usually curled nose to tail, facing the door behind us. The sense of the essence of his presence came slowly but, yes, it very definitely came. I believe the fact that Ed was still in his declining physical body, and that body was still unraveling, is what made the start of this reconnecting/reweaving gradual.

I didn't think of trying to "talk" with Ed, as if he'd just come home from work and I was calling out from the kitchen, "Hey there, did you have a good day?" I could sense his soul but I also sensed he was going through a tremendous amount, heavy duty stuff, most of it well beyond anything I could perceive or understand. It felt important just to be there in our familiar space for him, with him. I said the verse we'd always said together, read here and there in the various books we'd read together, hoping for an inner "ping!" of recognition or appreciation (there were a few faint "pings") then, during prayer time, asked if there was anything I could do for him. I wanted to be respectful about this, remembering how it had bothered him sometimes when folks said they were praying for him. He had heard those comments as expressions of pity, and he didn't want any of that. He wanted prayer — either his own prayers or those of others for him — to be an illuminative presence that could help him see his own way into his own relationship with the spiritual world. He was always clear on that.

So, I kept that wish of his in mind and envisioned light, sometimes white, sometimes gold, sometimes soft, other times bold and piercing, as a presence assisting him. There were days when I felt tension in him, inner stumbling akin to the outer physical PD stumbling, a close to desperate urge to climb out of his body, and numbing fatigue. With others, including my dad, I'd felt more removed, kind-of, "Well, he has to do it at his own pace," but with Ed my feeling was, "Golly, dying can be hard work!"

I remember watching *Call the Midwife* of Masterpiece Theater on TV the Sunday evening after Ed's birthday. Ed and I had watched it together for years and had enjoyed it. Each episode has several interwoven dramas which seem almost always to be more or less neatly resolved within the hour, yet there are a few unresolved questions to whet the appetite for the next installment. However, that Sunday, for the first time, I found the whole thing altogether unsatisfying. Because, when I turned the TV off, I felt I was returning to a really *awful* story playing out all around: the daily news, the rising number of COVID deaths, the forced separation from Ed, the fear, the loneliness. Tidy endings to movies: to heck with them! All I wanted was to go to bed and to sleep, to shoot far out into space, to get far away from it all.

Then, quite wonderfully, two nights later, I had the deepest dreamless sleep I'd had in months. I only woke once and was aware when I did wake — though very briefly — of being surrounded by protective figures. There were four, two of whom were friends on the other side. No words or thoughts were exchanged, they were simply there beside me. It was wonderful to know I didn't have to be on watch, I could go back where I'd been and get more of the delicious sleep, and off I went. I was deeply moved by the presence of these figures, had never sensed them in this way before, and named them my Sleep Guards or Sleep Sentries. I mention them because I was reassured that, not only were they there when I needed them, Ed also—indeed *everyone*—has their own Sleep Sentries whether they're ever aware of them or not. And actually not just at night, any time. There *are* beings in the invisible realms who care about us and what's happening here on earth.

When Christa called the unit for updates six or so days after Ed had been admitted, she was told he was unresponsive but not unconscious. I wasn't surprised considering how incoherent he looked on FaceTime but was puzzled by "unresponsive but not unconscious." Don't you have to be conscious to respond outwardly? Maybe what they were saying was that he wasn't in a vegetative state because he was still taking fluids and eating a little bit. And it was, frankly, hard to imagine Ed *not* eating after the enormous breakfast he'd downed the morning of the day after he returned from the nursing home. He'd always had a good, and a big, appetite, even when the pounds were melting off him because of the PD. He actually worried about getting a pot belly while making new notches on his belt so he could pull it in tighter. I teased him about that whenever I realized all the ice cream in the freezer had disappeared. All the yogurt popsicles too.

Though I was still inclined not to try to talk directly with Ed during our morning time, I wrote him several letters. We had corresponded for a year after we first met, when he was abroad teaching in Lebanon and I was working at Yale, and really met one another in thought and heart during that time by way of handwritten letters. Now, unable to talk with him in person—he was in a way abroad—I resorted again to the written word. I needed to express the profound thanks I felt for him giving me such a wonderful home in his heart. After trying to express that, I told him I'd taken my wedding band off and had put it in a safe place with his band. I explained that, as far as I was concerned, he was free to go on and I was certain, though I would miss him greatly, I would be okay. This seemed important not just because he'd always been protective of me—in fact, the name Edward means Guardian—but because I had once years earlier felt the anguish of a father on the other side who worried about his wife and children and how they were going to manage without him. What I had had to learn about legal and financial management and insurance after my father died had prepared me to some extent for what would come. And, though I'm oblivious to most of the rattles in the car, or smoke alarms when asleep, or strangers at the back door, or coyotes out in the field, I'd decided early on in my life, even before I met Ed, that I'd somehow find ways to hear what I needed to hear. That, so far, has been the case. And dog ears have always assisted me and kept me well informed!

The girls also had their own intuitions as to how it was going for Ed, and those tender knowings, though not quite as specific as mine (as, for example, in connection with his physical fatigue and his emotional regrets) called forth love, hope and deep sympathy for him. I am certain their responses meant a huge amount to him. In short, though there was, for them (and me too) an open, ongoing ache of loss, they wanted what was best for him, above what they wished they could get for themselves (meaning a physically present father and grandfather). It was also at this point that I became aware of something that continues even now: the grief that comes and goes in waves, isn't ours alone, it's Ed's too. We are still interwoven. We are feeling his grief over separation, even as he is feeling our missing him.

I know the date we learned Ed had contacted COVID—April 14th—but various things are jumbled in my memory. I think this is because my focus was much more on my inner connection with Ed which wasn't bound to time in the same way as outer events were. Put another way, I can't remember if my experience of the Sleep Sentries came before or after we heard about the COVID. I didn't write about that experience or other similar early hour happenings in my journal while moving between waking and sleeping. (Doubt I could even hold a pen at that hour.) Such experiences can be intense when they occur and can fade into the background quickly in the glare of everyday thinking. Outwardly you have facts to back you up when you're remembering something. With inner experiences, you remember the power of the emotional impact, and that may change how you think about the world, but how can you convince others of this power if they haven't experienced it themselves? For me it's an ongoing dilemma.

In terms of outer events, I remember we were shocked, yet not altogether shocked, by the diagnosis. We knew COVID was spreading far more rapidly where Ed was than where we were. The hospital Ed had been moved to actually tracked back to our local hospital to figure out where he might have first been exposed to COVID. I was questioned too but wasn't tested because the researchers concluded he'd caught it in the psychiatric unit. I was impressed by the thoroughness of these researchers and their determination to contain the virus.

At first I was upset because the COVID diagnosis meant Ed would have to be moved yet again and that would mean another hospital, another new doctor, new nurses and likely less intimate care because of masks, gloves, gowns, et cetera. But Ed was so much elsewhere, in this "unresponsive yet not unconscious" stage, those things didn't matter that much. Best of all, Ed had a truly wonderful doctor. This young Hispanic man made a point of asking for me several times on FaceTime because he kept hearing Ed saying my name. This was a gift to me because, I took it to mean I <u>was</u> reaching and connecting with Ed inwardly. It was similar to, yet not exactly the same as, the moment I shared earlier when my father was talking about me.

Dr. D (I regret I now can't find his name) explained that the low grade fever Ed had could stay level, then taper off, or, within three to five days, worsen dramatically. He said the virus was unpredictable and not to be complacent because the temperature was low. When I asked him how *he* was doing, he said he'd never in his life seen so many people stricken all at once and so many people dying so rapidly day after day. And how he hoped he would never have to witness anything like this again down the road. It meant a lot to me that, even if on the front lines and in constant demand at all hours, this doctor took the time to step aside, lower his mask very briefly so I could read his lips, and talk with me. He was heroic. I was so grateful Ed was with him.

Then Ed developed a cough which indicated pneumonia and things *did* move rapidly within three days...

It came to me early one morning before the COIVID spiraled downwards that Ed needed some inner assistance. There was this feeling of inner "stuck-ness" that reminded me of the physical "stuck-ness" Ed had displayed in March when he first went to the hospital ER and I knew I'd reached the end of being able to care for him physically.

But, as I couldn't see this situation with inner eyes the way I'd been able to see Ed struggling in his rigid body, I contacted one of my spiritual 911 numbers: my long-time friend and mentor, David Spangler. David listened, consulted his inner colleagues, then said I needed to become the portal through which Ed could step out of his body and move on into his next chapter. David added I would know what to do and how to do it

My first response to David's words was disbelief. Did I even know *what* he was talking about? I doubted it, but the confidence he had expressed gave me pause. And, when I paused, I realized I *did* have a sense of the way to go. It was deep in me. Furthermore, the way I would go would probably not have been the way David would have gone. Meaning, we really have to find our own way within ourselves. And now to help Ed find his own way.

I used a meditation Ed and I had done mostly alone, each of us on our own, now and then. It was familiar and dear to both of us. Its structure has been described many times by David in his writings and workshops and both Ed and I had adapted it to suit ourselves. The core of this meditation is called the Standing Exercise.

To describe roughly what I did: I sat in the chair I always use during the morning time imagining Ed, in his chair to my right. After being quiet for a few minutes I stood, eyes closed, inwardly seeing Ed also rising to stand beside me.

We were facing south. I spoke aloud, offering thanks first for our physical bodies and the fact that we could stand upright. Then thanks for the fact that Ed and I had met and shared so many years together. Followed by thanks for our families, our parents and brothers, our children, their children, close friends, colleagues, and others, all also standing.

Then Ed and I turned, facing west, eyes still closed. Still speaking aloud, I offered thanks for the Earth, its beauty and its bounty, the seasons, the mineral, plant and animal kingdoms, the winds, waters, and more.

Next we faced north and I gave thanks for the times into which we had incarnated and historical highlights and challenges that came to mind. These particular thanks –ending with thanks for COVID *and* PD—were harder for me to express. I ended that list with a quote I'd found in one of Brian Doyle's books:

We are part of a Mystery we do not understand and we are grateful.

Then we turned and faced east. I got the strong inner impression of a path opening up before us. We'd hiked together for years, up and down many mountains in different parts of the United States and abroad, but I knew this path was just for Ed. It was truly time for us to part. First I expressed thanks for the sun, the moon, the stars and the many celestial beings around and out there overseeing this path. Then, without looking in Ed's direction, keeping my eyes on this path, I thanked Ed again, said I looked forward to meeting with him again, and wished him Godspeed on his journey.

He moved forwards. I saw his back, then I couldn't see him anymore.

Ed stopped eating and remained unresponsive but not unconscious. I knew from experiences with others that one can hang on or stay around for a while after the appetite goes.

In the early morning of the day after the meditation, I had a dream in which I was looking through some stuff upstairs in our house. I carried a bundle of clothes downstairs to sort through on the dining room table and, as I put it all down, out jumped a fairly large and beautiful orange marmalade cat!

My first thought was, "Gosh, it could have suffocated in there!" (In the pile of clothes.)

The cat ran out an open door and off into the distance.

I've never thought of Ed as being like a cat, but do believe we all have "catness" — a bold, independent, wild streak within—and it can be imperative at times for our survival.

The overall feeling of that dream was release.

Christa called on FaceTime later that morning in tears. Dr. D said everything was speeding up: higher fever, difficulty breathing, nagging cough. Shortly after that call, Christa called again to say Dr. D wanted to know if it was okay for Ed to go on morphine. I said yes right away. He repeated that Ed's going might take a couple of days, but because of the PD it might take less time.

Later Christa called yet again to ask about connecting with Hospice. My first thought was, "For whom?" Things seemed to be moving so rapidly, did it matter? Would it be helpful for the girls? Did *I* need it? I didn't think so but…? The girls persuaded me to connect with Hospice, pointing out that it would mean their father would have someone with him at his bedside, and the organization could help us figure out what needed to be done after Ed passed over.

That afternoon I looked out the window and there was Ed's dear friend, Leslie, dressed in a bright orange sweatshirt, very similar to the color of the orange marmalade cat in my dream! Leslie had felt compelled to come to walk round our gardens and our yard as he'd done many times over the years with Ed.

After Leslie left, I knew *I* had to go walking too, with Tucker, to Wilcox Hollow, the spot by the Deerfield River, where Ed had loved to fish and later to sit and meditate. You can drive down a steep, bumpy dirt road to this spot or walk down by way of a path through the woods. I chose the path through a forest of red pine then along a bluff overseeing the river, though Ed hadn't been on it for about a year.

The spring run-off was *very* high, *very* active. I could actually hear it thundering from where I was high up. Down on the stony shore, Tucker and I stood beside the swirling waters for a while then made our way back up the bluff.

Going up I suddenly felt weak, as though everything—pathway, trees, rocks, earth, Tucker and I, *everything*—could be swept away. The vitality of the river, the raw force of it, was scary. But, as I reached the top of the bluff I began to feel lighter and lighter, as though a great load was being lifted off my shoulders and I hadn't realized how heavy it was.

Two days later in a waking dream, I heard the thundering again. It was a roar of something coming closer and closer. Then I saw swirling waters again—hurtling and churning onwards—and saw, with horror and some fear, human figures being tossed into the air. They tumbled down in the waves, then up again like rag dolls, then down again. With this came the sense of *many*—not just Ed—going over. It felt as though I was seeing a picture of the pandemic.

Then I saw that there were, in the midst of all this, some upright figures who were on what looked like paddle boards, surfboards, or shafts of light. They were balancing and riding the wild waves. I was relieved by the feeling that I *wasn't* seeing a scene of total chaos and destruction.

When I woke from this dream, there was the certainty: Ed was upright and on his way!

About three hours later, when lying on the sofa in the living room half-awake, half- napping, a sound on the window beside the sofa, jolted me awake. As I scrambled to my knees on the sofa and looked out, a large bird with a red spot on its head– a Flicker—flew very close to the living room window pane. It did this twice, without crashing against the glass, hovering in the air, as though looking into the house.

I have, several times, had experiences with birds right before someone I know has died. To me they were messengers, so I wasn't startled. But a woodpecker? Ed was, I thought then, no more like a woodpecker than a marmalade cat.

Sometime later, after Ed has passed over, our grandson gave me an old Christmas tree ornament that he loved, a wooden woodpecker with a red spot on its head. And I *was* startled then, because Wynn didn't know about the bird I'd seen at the window. As I held the ornament in my hands I had to smile as the thought came to me, "Ed who loved wood and wood turning and woodcarving sure *was* something of a *wood pecker*!"

Christa was with me when Hospice was called in and took all the phone calls from them. The night of the day when the woodpecker looked in the house was the first time a Hospice nurse sat beside Ed.

I can't remember if the nurse was with him all night, only remember that I went early the next morning to the grocery store while Christa took off for a quick run on the hill. And when I returned around 7:30, a full bag of groceries in both arms, Christa met me at the back door. It was clear, from one look at her face, Ed had gone on.

Shortly After the Passing

All three of us—Laurel, Christa and I—felt tremendous relief from Ed, very soon after his passing. Relief that he was at last free of his body. We can't prove any of this, yet the sameness of our inner impressions of Ed, even when we're not together, when we're involved in our very different lives at a distance, even now months later, feels like proof to us, proof that it's possible to connect with those who have passed over. There have been days when I've felt blue about Ed having to experience such an isolated, inelegant death—he couldn't even be in his own clothing.

Laurel or Christa, sometimes both together, have often spontaneously emailed to share the sadness they're feeling. And there have been days when we've found ourselves humming or singing the songs that became Ed's exhaling during his last year and a half. And we share our sense of him often offering us suggestions, "Go there…" "Read that…" "Be in touch with so-and-so…."

We connected with a funeral home which made arrangements with the hospital, both girls contacted family and friends near and far, Laurel wrote an obituary and helped put together a memorial card since it was clear we wouldn't be able to offer a memorial service because of the virus. We did have a brief eventide service at home one evening a few nights after Ed died with one of the ministers of the church I, and sometimes Ed, occasionally attended. Then both girls returned to their families—Christa going east first to the hospital where Ed had died to pick up his personal belongings, then west to her own home.

Early in May the girls and their husbands, children and dogs returned for a long week-end. We all wanted, indeed needed, to be together to talk, hug, cry, laugh and create our own impromptu service for Ed.

A day or two before the children arrived, I woke around 3:00

am and "saw" Ed in the doorway of our bedroom. He was standing there, hands on the door frame, the way he had sometimes rested briefly at that very spot before making the final trek from bathroom, through the hallway, to his side of the bed. I couldn't see his face, as the only light was from the bathroom some distance behind him. But I got up instantly, thinking he needed help, and—he was gone when I reached the door. Four hours later I received an email that his ashes had arrived in town, and could I please pick them up? Not having been notified by the funeral home as to when the ashes would reach us, I thanked Ed for letting me know he would be present physically, as well as in spirit, at our family gathering.

Food, flowers, cards, letters, and emails were arriving daily and continued to come for months afterwards. I was astonished—still am—by the outpouring of sympathy, empathy, love, grief, gratitude and memories. Students, friends and former colleagues of Ed's from up to 55 years ago have reached out unexpectedly and asked to reconnect. And the words they all use sound like a series of ongoing refrains in a song: how closely Ed listened, how interested he was in others, how kind, thoughtful and sometimes mischievous! The fact that we couldn't have a church service even now makes these communications feel as though we—and Ed—are standing in the midst of an *ongoing* service. And I can hear and see Ed's amazement and bafflement: "Why all the fuss?" "What did I do... I really didn't do much." "Why *me*?"

Our family gathered in the living room of our house in the early morning of Sunday May 3, close to the time Ed had passed over. I'd made a paper prayer flag of photos of Ed, photos that had been taken over the years with each one of us with him, also a few of all of us together, and taped the flag to the mantelpiece. There were other photos around the room of him as a child, teenager, and young man, him at work, and with his brothers, his mother, my parents, and our wider families. There were flowers from the garden on the mantelpiece, along with a row of bowls Ed had turned on the lathe. His ashes were in the middle bowl, made of cherry.

Everyone had gone upstairs the afternoon before to see if there was any clothing in Ed's closet they wanted, and *everyone* had taken something: a shirt or a sweater, a necktie or pair of socks. We were a motley crew with two granddaughters in Ed's enormous bulky sweaters, the youngest granddaughter submerged in one of Ed's long-sleeved shirts that dragged on the floor like a floor mop and the one grandson in a familiar, fraying, everyday shirt Ed was totally comfortable in. I imagined Ed laughing at the distribution of his wardrobe, also surprised, even flattered, that the children wanted to draw close to the touch, feel and smell of what he'd worn. (The children continued to wear the items they'd picked whenever they felt like it, throughout the summer.)

Laurel, Christa and I sat on the sofa—the window where the Flicker had looked in behind us—the others gathered close around us and a table (which Ed had made) on which were candles. The central candle was for Ed, the others for each of us, including the three dogs.

After the candles had been lit, I told my story of meeting Ed and was amazed, as I talked, by the looks of total absorption on the faces of even the youngest usually *very* wiggly grandkids. We had prepared them in advance, informing them they could say anything they wanted about EBee—as they called him--and they did have memories to share. As did everyone else, in no set order, several adding on other memories later, all told from the heart, often with laughter and also with tears.

Next, we sang the songs that had befriended Ed during his last year and a half. Then, as the kids were beginning to squirm, we stepped outside into a beautiful warm day with the cherry bowl from the mantel, and the silver spoon that had been presented to Ed's grandparents on their 50th anniversary. We took turns spreading Ed's ashes around the trees, the rocks, the gardens, the fence…

Then, in the evening of that day, we all went to Wilcox Hollow. With Christa's help at the band saw, the kids had made little boats in Ed's wood shop. Everyone had a boat decorated in bright colors and/or with a message to Ed written on it. And we gave them all to the river.

A Year Later: April 2021

I find it quite mysterious how all that I have shared in this account can seem like a day or two ago and can also seem like a long, long time ago.

So, where is Ed a year later?

Until recently I've sensed him here, not only in this house but checking in with family and friends, with trees, rocks and rivers too. I was not surprised when, last February, I inwardly heard Ed suggesting I check the oil in the oil tank. I was grateful for that nudge as the tank was *very* low and a winter storm was coming. Nor have I been surprised when Laurel, Christa, or any one of the grandchildren, or any of Ed's good friends, either separately or all at once together, without knowing they are sounding the same note, have emailed to say they are aware of his presence.

I have seen Ed in dreams. In every one of them he does *not* have PD. It took me a while to get accustomed to this because of how bony, stooped and weak he was when I last saw him in his body. In the dreams he moves freely, easily, and looks quite a bit younger than I look. Ha! How dare he!

Right after April 19, 2021—the one year mark of his passing—I had a vivid dream. In this dream we were in a different house. This house was one floor, one large light-filled room, overlooking the ocean. The lines of the house were simple, clean, even elegant, in the vein of Frank Lloyd Wright whose architecture Ed much admired as a young man. Looking out the window I was amazed by what I saw: vast blue of water, white of air, gold of sun light; a meeting of earth and sky. Then Ed told me he wanted me to accompany him the next day on that ocean. He didn't say if by boat or where he might be going. He was excited to be going, and I was glad he was excited, but knew I couldn't go. I told him I was sorry, that I had several things to do (on land.) Then I looked out again at the ocean and saw the tide was coming in. I could see dark blue-black waves inching their way up the rocks down below… and…I woke up. The overall impression of the dream was of a changed, and rapidly changing, vista, not just for Ed, or for me, but for the whole world. And Ed and I had different things we needed to do, different ways to go. It was not a sad dream, it was an "on-we-go" dream.

Where am I a year later?

In all truthfulness, I'm not as excited about where I am, as Ed seemed to be in that dream about where he was going. I'm aware I still harbor anger at PD, anger at the destructive unraveling I witnessed up-close, and the forces of PD bearing down on others here whom I care about.

No, PD, I'm not through with you! But I can't fight you mind to mind, fist to fist the way the scientists are doing it—and God bless them in their efforts. I want to find ways to outwit you. Or—better yet—outlove you!
Outlove PD?
It's like this: I can't sugar-coat the PD experience, but I know, looking back over the 12 years Ed I and grappled with it, that Ed's love for life, and my love for life, and ours together, brought us more truly and deeply into this incarnation. And I am thankful for that.

I remember a day when a friend asked if the spiritual world was "helping" us –as if we had access to a private phone number we could call when we needed to know which way to go, what to do next, or simply to chat with God or some angel as to the meaning behind Ed's struggle and if it was worth it.

The question made me feel as though I was standing empty handed, in my most worn out clothes and sneakers on a seemingly endless hard, hot, flat road in the desert. I knew I had nothing to

78

share, nothing to show for where I was, and said the only thing I could think of, "The spiritual world? All I can say is that, right now, it's where the rubber hits the road."

I believe the "spiritual" world *is* where the rubber hits the road. By this I mean it's right here, not off on some distant mountain peak. It is *with* us wherever we may be, however we may chance or choose to begin to recognize, acknowledge, and work with it. This is where the reweaving occurs. As Ed unraveled, the spirit of love came to meet and reweave him –and me too— again and again, by way of children, friends, so many "right" people at the "right" moment, songs, dance, mime, poetry, dreams, intuitions, laughter, trees, bluebirds, starlight, and so much more.

No, I can't sugar-coat PD, or COVID-19 which, mercifully, took Ed when he needed and was ready to go on, but I can try to do all I can to keep the door open for love.

With Gratitude and Thanks

To Craig Latham, Lisa Murphy and Brian Maurer
for providing practical assistance and calm
during some major unraveling moments.

To Ruth Charney, Sister Joan, Leslie Luchonok,
Claude Pepin, Rob Mermin, Tom Yeomans,
who, by way of emails during the COVID lock-down,
kept me retrieving memories, weaving and reweaving all
into this account.

To Judith Quinn Blatchford
for cleaning up the crumbs.

To Jeremy Berg and David Spangler
for providing a home for this book.

CPSIA information can be obtained
at www.ICGtesting.com
Printed in the USA
BVHW041433160621
609642BV00005B/1353